Ophthalmic Research

Journal for Research in Experimental and Clinical Ophthalmology

Founded 1970 by O. Hockwin, Bonn, G. Naumann, Hamburg and D.F. Cole, London
Continued by O. Hockwin, Bonn, 1981–1994, G.F.J.M. Vrensen, Zeist, 1994–2003

KARGER

Printed in Switzerland
on acid-free and non-aging
paper (ISO 9706) by
Reinhardt Druck, Basel

Appears 6-weekly:
2 volumes per year
(8 issues)

Ophthalmic Research

Submission

Only original papers written in English are considered and should be submitted using the online submission website:

www.karger.com/ore

or as an e-mail attachment (the preferred word-processing package is MS-Word) to the Editorial Office:

Editorial Office 'Ophthalmic Research'
S. Karger AG
P.O. Box
CH-4009 Basel (Switzerland)
Tel +41 61 306 1356
Fax +41 61 306 1434
E-Mail ore@karger.ch

Types of Papers

(1) The main body of papers to be published will be *'Original Papers'* on experimental research. (2) *'Review Papers'* of up to 30 manuscript pages will be published from invited authors and by direct submission. In both cases the manuscripts will be subject to peer reviewing. Review papers will be published free of charge. (3) *'Mini Reviews'* of up to 10 manuscript pages (double-spaced, including an abstract of max. 200 words and references) should contain an easy-to-read literature overview on a specific topic. Papers are either invited or may be submitted for consideration. Please submit your mini review online. (4) *'Short Communications'* of up to 3–4 pages dealing with new original concepts or technical approaches will be published at short notice. (5) 'Ophthalmic Research' has a tradition in publishing *'Supplements'* which can be published under the responsibility of guest editors. Requests for such supplements should be addressed to the Editor-in-Chief.

Conditions

All manuscripts are subject to editorial review. Manuscripts are received with the explicit understanding that they are not under simultaneous consideration by any other publication except in abstract form. Submission of an article for publication implies transfer of the copyright from the author to the publisher upon acceptance. Accepted papers become the permanent property of 'Ophthalmic Research' and may not be reproduced by any means, in whole or in part, without the written consent of the publisher. It is the author's responsibility to obtain permission to reproduce illustrations, tables, etc. from other publications. Research involving live human and animal subjects must have been approved by the author's institutional review board. 'Ophthalmic Research' requires that in the Methods section of their manuscript the authors state that they adhered to the tenets of the Declaration of Helsinki or the NIH statement for the use of Animals in Research.

Conflicts of Interest

Authors are required to disclose any sponsorship or funding arrangements relating to their research and all authors should disclose any possible conflicts of interest. Conflict of interest statements will be published at the end of the article.

Arrangement

Title page: The first page of each paper should indicate the title, the authors' names, the institute where the work was conducted, and a short title for use as running head.

NB: Authors wishing to preserve the phonetic mean ing of diacritics (PubMed reduces diacritics to their root characters) must spell their names accordingly when submitting manuscripts (e.g. Müller should be Mueller).

Full address: The exact postal address of the corresponding author complete with postal code must be given at the bottom of the title page. Please also supply phone and fax numbers, as well as e-mail address.

Key words: For indexing purposes, a list of 3–10 key words in English is essential.

Abstract: Each paper needs an abstract of up to 10 lines.

Footnotes: Avoid footnotes.

Tables and illustrations: Tables and illustrations (both numbered in Arabic numerals) should be sent in separate files. Tables require a heading and figures a legend, also in a separate file. Due to technical reasons, figures with a screen background should not be submitted. When possible, group several illustrations in one block for reproduction (max. size 180 × 223 mm). Black and white half-tone and color illustrations must have a final resolution of 300 dpi after scaling, line drawings one of 800–1,200 dpi.

Color Illustrations
Online edition: Color illustrations are reproduced free of charge. In the print version, the illustrations are reproduced in black and white. Please avoid referring to the colors in the text and figure legends.
Print edition: Up to 6 color illustrations per page can be integrated within the text at CHF 800.– per page.

References: In the text identify references by Arabic numerals [in square brackets]. Material submitted for publication but not yet accepted should be noted as 'unpublished data' and not be included in the reference list. The list of references should include only those publications which are cited in the text. Do not alphabetize; number references in the order in which they are first mentioned in the text. The surnames of the authors followed by initials should be given. There should be no punctuation other than a comma to separate the authors. Preferably, please cite all authors. Abbreviate journal names according to the Index Medicus system. (Also see International Committee of Medical Journal Editors: Uniform requirements for manuscripts submitted to biomedical journals. N Engl J Med 1997;336:309–315. www.icmje.org).

Examples
(a) Papers published in periodicals: Chatel J-M, Bernard H, Orson FM: Isolation and characterization of two complete Ara h 2 isoforms cDNA. Int Arch Allergy Immunol 2003;131:14–18.
(b) Papers published only with DOI numbers: Theoharides TC, Boucher W, Spear K: Serum interleukin-6 reflects disease severity and osteoporosis in mastocytosis patients. Int Arch Allergy Immunol DOI: 10.1159/000063858.
(c) Monographs: Matthews DE, Farewell VT: Using and Understanding Medical Statistics, ed 3, revised. Basel, Karger, 1996.
(d) Edited books: DuBois RN: Cyclooxygenase-2 and colorectal cancer; in Dannenberg AJ, Dubois RN (eds): COX-2. Prog Exp Tum Res. Basel, Karger, 2003, vol 37, pp 124–137.

Reference Management Software: Use of EndNote is recommended for easy management and formatting of citations and reference lists.

Digital Object Identifier (DOI)

S. Karger Publishers supports DOIs as unique identifiers for articles. A DOI number will be printed on the title page of each article. DOIs can be useful in the future for identifying and citing articles published online without volume or issue information. More information can be found at www.doi.org.

Author's Choice™

Karger's Author's Choice service broadens the reach of your article and gives all users worldwide free and full access for reading, downloading and printing at www.Karger.com. The option is available for a one-time fee of CHF 3000.–, which is a permissible cost in grant allocation. More information can be found at www.karger.com/authors_choice.

NIH-Funded Research

The U.S. National Institutes of Health (NIH) mandates under the NIH Public Access Policy that final, peer-reviewed manuscripts appear in its digital database within 12 months of the official publication date. As a service to authors, Karger submits the final version of your article on your behalf to PubMed Central. For those selecting our premium Author's Choice service, we will send your article immediately upon publishing, accelerating the accessibility of your work without the usual embargo. More details on NIH's Public Access Policy is available at http://publicaccess.nih.gov/FAQ.htm#a1

Self-Archiving

Karger permits authors to archive their pre-prints (i.e. pre-refereeing) or post-prints (i.e. final draft post-refereeing) on their personal or institution's servers, provided the following conditions are met: Articles may not be used for commercial purposes, must be linked to the publisher's version, and must acknowledge the publisher's copyright. Authors selecting Karger's Author's Choice feature, however, are also permitted to archive the final, published version of their article, which includes copyediting and design improvements as well as citation links.

Page Charges

There are no page charges for papers of 3 or fewer printed pages (including tables, illustrations and references). Each additional complete or partial page is charged to the author at CHF 650.–. The allotted size of a paper is equal to approx. 8 double-spaced manuscript pages (including abstract, tables, illustrations and references).

Proofs

Unless indicated otherwise, proofs are sent to the first-named author and should be returned with the least possible delay. Alterations made in proofs, other than the correction of printer's errors, are charged to the author. No page proofs are supplied.

Reprints

Order forms and a price list are sent with the proofs. Orders submitted after the issue is printed are subject to considerably higher prices.

KARGER

Fax +41 61 306 12 34
E-Mail karger@karger.ch
www.karger.com

The Guidelines for Authors are available at:
www.karger.com/ore_Guidelines

General Information

Ophthalmic Research

ISSN Print Edition: 0030–3747
ISSN Online Edition: 1423–0259

Journal Homepage: www.karger.com/ore

Publication Data: 'Ophthalmic Research' is published 8 times a year. Volumes 43, 44, each with 4 issues, appear in 2010.

Subscription Rates: Subscriptions run for a full calendar year. Prices are given per year.

Personal subscription:

Print or Online	**Print+Online combined**
CHF 862.–	CHF 952.–
EUR 616.–	EUR 680.–
USD 782.00	USD 868.00

postage and handling (added to print and print+online)
CHF 50.40 Europe, CHF 75.60 Overseas
EUR 36.–
USD 71.60

Institutional subscription:

Print or Online	**Print+Online combined**
CHF 1724.–	CHF 1896.–
EUR 1232.–	EUR 1354.–
USD 1564.00	USD 1720.00

postage and handling (added to print and print+online)
CHF 63.20 Europe, CHF 94.40 Overseas
EUR 44.80
USD 89.60

Airmail surcharge: CHF 64.– / USD 60.80

Discount subscription prices:
- European Association for Visim and Eye Research (EVER)
- Association for Research and Vision in Ophthalmology (ARVO)

Back Volumes and Single Issues: Information on availability and prices of single print issues and print or electronic back volumes can be obtained from Customer Service at *service@karger.ch.*

Bibliographic Indices: This journal is regularly listed in bibliographic services, including *Current Contents®* and PubMed/MEDLINE.

Photocopying: This journal has been registered with the Copyright Clearance Center (CCC), as indicated by the code appearing on the first page of each article. For readers in the US, this code signals consent for copying of articles for personal or internal use, or for the personal or internal use of specific clients, provided that the stated fee is paid per copy directly to
Copyright Clearance Center Inc.
222 Rosewood Drive
Danvers, MA 01923 (USA)
A copy of the first page of the article must accompany payment. Consent does not extend to copying for general distribution, for promotion, for creating new works, or for resale. In these cases, specific written permission must be obtained from the copyright owner,
S. Karger AG, P.O. Box
CH–4009 Basel (Switzerland).

Subscription Orders:
Orders can be placed at agencies, bookstores, directly with the Publisher

S. Karger AG
Medical and Scientific Publishers
P.O. Box
CH–4009 Basel
Switzerland
(for courier services only:
Allschwilerstrasse 10
CH–4055 Basel)
Tel. +41 61 306 11 11
Fax +41 61 306 12 34
E-Mail karger@karger.ch
www.karger.com

or further Karger offices or representatives:

France:
Librairie Medi-Sciences Sarl
36, bd de Latour-Maubourg
75007 Paris
France
Tél. +33 (0) 1 45 51 42 58
Fax +33 (0) 1 45 56 07 80
E-Mail librairie@medi-sciences.fr
www.medi-sciences.fr

Germany:
S. Karger GmbH
Postfach
79095 Freiburg
Deutschland
(Hausadresse: Wilhelmstrasse 20 A
79098 Freiburg)
Tel. +49 761 45 20 70
Fax +49 761 45 20 714
E-Post information@karger.de
www.karger.de

India, Bangladesh, Sri Lanka:
Panther Publishers Private Ltd.
33, First Main
Koramangala First Block
Bangalore 560 034
India
Tel. +91 80 25505 836
Tel. +91 80 25505 837
Fax +91 80 25505 981
E-Mail panther_publishers@vsnl.com
www.pantherpublishers.com

Japan:
Karger Japan, Inc.
Yushima S Bld. 3F
4-2-3, Yushima, Bunkyo-ku
Tokyo 113-0034
Japan
Tel. +81 3 3815 1800
Fax +81 3 3815 1802
E-Mail publisher@karger.jp

China, Taiwan and Malaysia:
Karger China
Suite 409, Apollo Building
1440 Central Yan An Road
Shanghai 200040
China
Tel. +86-21-6133 1861
Fax +86-21-6133 1862
E-Mail karger.ray@gmail.com

South America and Central America:
Cranbury International LLC
7 Clarendon Ave., Suite 2
Montpelier, VT 05602
USA
Tel. +1 802 223 6565
Fax +1 802 223 6824
E-Mail
eatkin@cranburyinternational.com
www.cranburyinternational.com

United Kingdom, Ireland:
S. Karger AG
c/o London Liaison Office
4 Rickett Street
London SW6 1RU
United Kingdom
Tel. +44 (0) 20 7386 0500
Fax +44 (0) 20 7610 3337
E-Mail uk@karger.ch

USA:
S. Karger Publishers, Inc.
26 West Avon Road
P.O. Box 529
Unionville, CT 06085
USA
Toll free: +1 800 828 5479
Tel. +1 860 675-7834
Fax +1 860 675-7302
E-Mail karger@snet.net

Change of Address:
Both old and new address should be sent to the subscription source.

KARGER

Fax +41 61 306 12 34
E-Mail karger@karger.ch
www.karger.com

The Journal Home Page is available at:
www.karger.com/ore

Ophthalmic Research

Anti-Aging in Ophthalmology

Guest Editor

Kazuo Tsubota, Tokyo

20 figures, 2 in color, and 5 tables, 2010

KARGER Basel · Freiburg · Paris · London · New York · Bangalore · Bangkok · Shanghai · Singapore · Tokyo · Sydney

S. Karger
Medical and Scientific Publishers
Basel • Freiburg • Paris • London •
New York • Bangalore • Bangkok •
Shanghai • Singapore • Tokyo • Sydney

P.O. Box, CH–4009 Basel (Switzerland)
Printed in Switzerland
on acid-free and non-aging paper (ISO 9706) by
Reinhardt Druck, Basel
ISBN 978–3–8055–9574–2
e-ISBN 978–3–8055–9575–9

KARGER

Fax +41 61 306 12 34
E-Mail karger@karger.ch
www.karger.com

Vol. 44, No. 3, 2010

Ophthalmic Research

Contents

KARGER

Fax +41 61 306 12 34
E-Mail karger@karger.ch
www.karger.com

Access to full text and tables of contents, including tentative ones for forthcoming issues: www.karger.com/ore_issues

Ophthalmic Research

Ophthalmic Res 2010;44:145
DOI: 10.1159/000316446

Published online: September 9, 2010

Editorial

The life span in developed countries has been increasing for the last 20 years, and surprisingly this trend is likely to continue its steady increase over the upcoming decades too. The impact of this trend is that the population consists of more elderly people. Since elderly people show a tendency towards age-related eye disorders, modern societies are transferring this major challenge to the ophthalmic community. The major blinding diseases such as cataracts, glaucoma, diabetic retinopathy and age-related macular degeneration are most affected by aging. Even the genetic disorders, such as retinitis pigmentosa, can be considered 'premature aging of the retina' and are affected by aging. Not only the blinding diseases, but also other major diseases such as dry eye or presbyopia, which dramatically affect quality of vision, are affected by aging. Thus, in the aging societies of developed countries, aging is a very important factor in ophthalmology.

Recent advances in the understanding of aging have given us a new way of thinking about the intervention in the aging process. The advances in aging research may be able to provide the chance to interfere with the aging process itself, including that of the eye. One hard evidence comes from calorie restriction (CR) intervention. CR extends the life span in many species. Fortunately CR can also suppress the incidence of age-related diseases such as cancer, diabetes and cardiovascular events, and possibly age-related eye disorders.

In addition to the CR theory, the oxidative stress theory is another important hypothesis that is believed to be involved in aging. According to this theory, we can manage the aging process by controlling reactive oxygen species (ROS). Since the main function of the eye is 'seeing' which is mediated by photoprocessing of the retinal cells, light exposure, especially blue to ultraviolet light, can induce ROS. The production of ROS in the retina is an unavoidable event of normal eye function. Also, the ocular surface is exposed to the ambient environment of which oxygen levels fluctuate with each blink and polluted air. Thus, the ROS theory is also a very important consideration.

In this issue focusing on the antiaging approach for eye disorders, there are reviews based on the CR theory and the oxidative stress theory. The first review by Tsubota et al. for dry eye care is based on the two aforementioned theories. The CR-theory-based reviews in this issue point out the importance of mitochondria (paper by Jarrett et al.) and sirtuins (article by Ozawa and Kubota). These issues provide new challenges and are expected to open a very important field in the near future. The oxidative-stress-theory-based reviews comprise evidence from epidemiological studies (by Fletcher), the importance of nutrition (by Agte and Tarwadi), prevention of age-related cataracts (by Beebe et al.) and glaucoma (by Chrysostomou et al.). These reviews offer new and comprehensive information; thus, the readers can obtain a clear picture on how the oxidative control is important for the prevention and treatment of eye diseases from the point of view of aging.

Antiaging research has recently come of age. The practical approach using the fundamentals of aging research is not used clinically yet; however, ROS control, such as supplementation based on the Age-Related Eye Disease Study, is the beginning of the application of ROS control for the age-related disorders. A proper diet, including CR or antioxidant food factors, antioxidant supplements and exercise may become important interventions for the age-related eye disorders. Future developments may include drug intervention in addition to supplements based on the antiaging approach.

Kazuo Tsubota, Tokyo

KARGER

Fax +41 61 306 12 34
E-Mail karger@karger.ch
www.karger.com

0030–3747/10/0443–0145$26.00/0

Accessible online at:
www.karger.com/ore

Ophthalmic Research

Ophthalmic Res 2010;44:146–154
DOI: 10.1159/000316594

Published online: September 9, 2010

The Era of Antiaging Ophthalmology Comes of Age: Antiaging Approach for Dry Eye Treatment

Kazuo Tsubota[a] Motoko Kawashima[a] Takaaki Inaba[a] Murat Dogru[a] Yoko Ogawa[a] Shigeru Nakamura[a] Ken Shinmura[b] Akihiro Higuchi[a] Tetsuya Kawakita[a]

Departments of [a]Ophthalmology and [b]Internal Medicine, Keio University School of Medicine, Tokyo, Japan

Key Words

Aging · Dry eye · Calorie restriction · Reactive oxygen species

Abstract

Recent advances in the understanding of aging have paved a new way of thinking about intervening with the aging process. There is a global agreement in the scientific community that calorie restriction (CR) can actually extend the life span of various kinds of animals so that this has become a real intervention in aging. In addition to the CR theory, the free radical theory is another important hypothesis, which is believed to be involved in aging. According to this theory, we can manage the aging process by controlling calories or reactive oxygen species. In this paper, these two important aging theories, CR and free radical aging, are reviewed, and it is discussed how to apply these theories to the prevention and treatment of eye diseases. Finally, we share the preliminary results of our animal study on dry eye, and I report my personal experience as a dry eye patient, which has been alleviated by the *antiaging approach*.

Introduction

There has been a rapid increase in dry eye patients around the world. The reason has yet to be elucidated, but the spread of visual display terminal use, longer working hours, shortened sleeping time, increase in stress level, environmental factors and increased life span are considered to be at least part of the reason for the increase in dry eye patients. Even high school students have shown a high incidence of dry eye syndrome although the incidence in older people is far higher [1–3]. Among visual display terminal workers in Japan, the incidence of dry eye is almost 22% in women and over 10% in men, (1) which means there are potentially more than 24 million dry eye patients in Japan. Among them, aging is one of the most important factors for the pathogenesis of dry eye. It is well known that dry eye occurs less often in children and that people lose tear function with age [4]. We have recently reported that 73% of the elderly population exhibit dry eye syndrome, which was far more than expected [3]. In ophthalmology, there are many age-related diseases such as cataract, macular degeneration, glaucoma, pterygium, conjunctival chalasis,

KARGER

Fax +41 61 306 12 34
E-Mail karger@karger.ch
www.karger.com

0030–3747/10/0443–0146$26.00/0

Accessible online at:
www.karger.com/ore

Kazuo Tsubota
Department of Ophthalmology
Keio University School of Medicine
35 Shinanomachi, Shinjuku-ku, Tokyo 160-8582 (Japan)
Tel. +81 3 5363 3269, Fax +81 3 3358 5961, E-Mail tsubota@sc.itc.keio.ac.jp

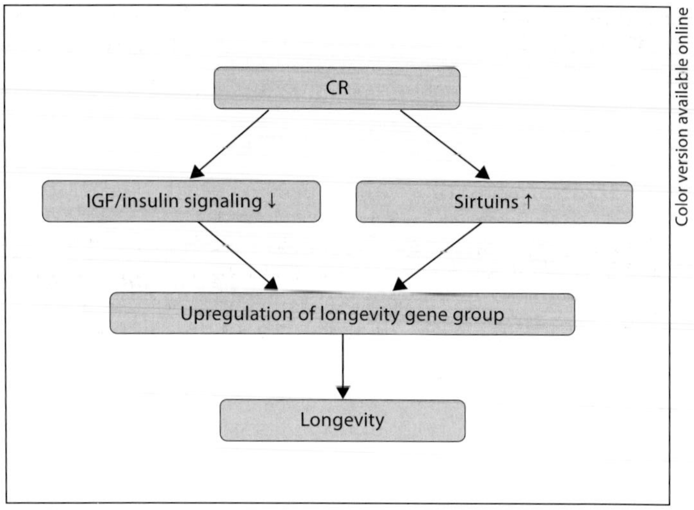

Fig. 1. CR decreases the insulin-like growth factor (IGF)/insulin signaling and increases sirtuin activity, resulting in various kinds of gene upregulation associated with longevity.

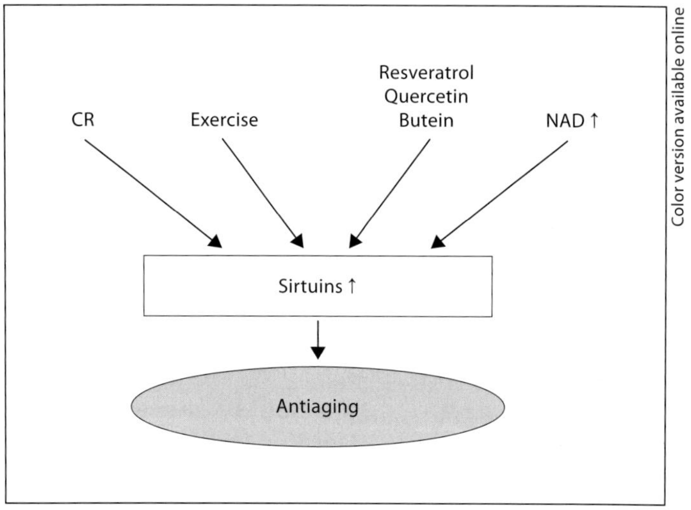

Fig. 2. The effects of sirtuin on the various longevity-related aspects.

diabetic retinopathy, retinal vein occlusion and senile ptosis in addition to dry eye, which counts for more than 80% of all the eye diseases. Thus, aging is an important risk factor for eye diseases.

Recent advances in the understanding of aging have provided a new way of thinking about intervention in the aging process. It had been considered that the aging process was so complex that we could not intervene until the total view of aging could be understood. However, there is a global agreement in the scientific community that calorie restriction (CR) can extend the life span in various kinds of animals so that this has become a true intervention in the aging process [5, 6]. The important point about CR is that it also suppresses the incidence of age-related diseases such as cancer, diabetes and/or cardiovascular events. According to the CR theory, we can postpone age-related diseases or even treat age-related diseases by total CR or mimetics of CR [5]. This is a remarkable advancement in aging science in that we declare that we can interfere with aging with antiaging strategies today. In addition to the CR theory, the free radical theory is another important hypothesis which is believed to be involved in aging [7]. According to this theory, we can manage the aging process by controlling reactive oxygen species (ROS).

In this paper, we would like to review these two important aging theories, CR and free radical aging, and to discuss how to apply these theories for the prevention and treatment of eye diseases. Finally, we share the preliminary results of our animal study in dry eye and I (K.T.) report my personal experience as a dry eye patient.

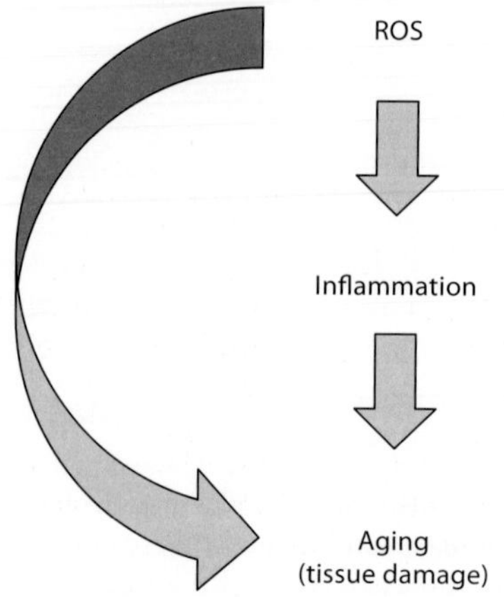

Color version available online

Fig. 3. ROS induce many changes in lipids, proteins and DNA, resulting in aging, as well as produce inflammation which contributes to the aging process.

CR Theory

The average and maximum life span of many species – from yeast and nematodes to rodents and monkeys – can be increased by up to 50% by reducing calorie intake compared with *ad libitum* food intake [5]. As reported by microarray analysis, CR affects the gene expression patterns during aging and provides for a healthier life [8]. Some molecular mechanisms of the effect of CR are becoming clear such as the suppression of insulin-like growth factor/insulin signaling or activation of sirtuin molecules (fig. 1) [9, 10].

CR also reduces the incidence of age-related diseases such as cancer, cardiovascular disease and immune dysfunction [11–13]. As a consequence, the physiological changes caused by CR contribute towards a better health condition and provide greater longevity [13]. Since the CR lifestyle is difficult to follow in daily life, vigorous efforts are being undertaken to seek an alternative of CR by producing the same molecular effect in the body [14–16], by CR mimetics. Possible CR mimetic products include various kinds of polyphenols such as resveratrol, quercetin and butein [14]. Resveratrol upregulates the activity and transcription of sirtuins, thus providing the beneficial effect. Consequently activation of sirtuins interacts with various transcriptional molecules (fig. 2), resulting in the expression and maintenance of the antiaging effect [17, 18]. Thus, many pharmaceutical companies are now searching for better molecules of CR mimetics for the prevention and treatment of diseases.

In humans, it is clear that chronic high calorie intake over time is a risk factor in various age-related diseases as observed in metabolic syndrome [19]. It is not yet clear whether age-related eye diseases are also prevented by CR, but this seems highly possible and could be a great intervention in important blinding diseases [20–22]. According to the CR theory, aging and age-related diseases can be controlled by the simple concept of CR.

Free Radical Theory

The free radical aging hypothesis was first proposed by Harman [7] in 1956 and has been considered to be the major mechanism of aging (fig. 3). The free radical theory or ROS, used almost interchangeably, attack the important cell molecules of proteins, lipids and DNA. ROS are generated in the mitochondria, cytoplasm and extracellular components. The overproduction of ROS in the mitochondria shortens the nematode life span [23]. In contrast, overexpression of superoxide dismutase (SOD) and catalase, which are antioxidant enzymes, can increase the life span of *Drosophila* or the mouse [24, 25]. Among them, ROS generated by the mitochondria are considered to be the major type, but the photoinduced ROS are not negligible. In dermatology, the aging of the skin is considered to be caused mainly by light, called photoaging. In photoaging, ROS are the major players. Since light and ultraviolet light exposures are the important risk factors for cataract as well as age-related macular

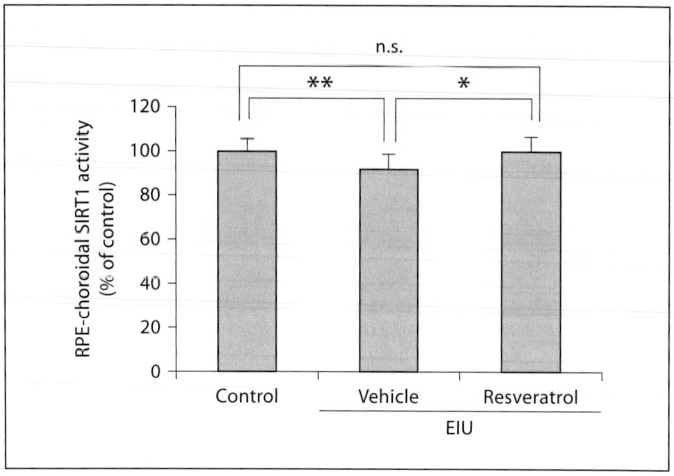

Fig. 4. Activation of sirtuin (SIRT1) by resveratrol in the choroid. Retinal pigment epithelium (RPE)-choroidal SIRT1 activities were significantly ($p < 0.01$) lower in vehicle-treated endotoxin-induced uveitis (EIU) mice than in vehicle-treated controls. Systemic administration of resveratrol (50 mg/kg body weight) to endotoxin-induced uveitis animals led to a significant ($p < 0.05$) increase in SIRT1 activity in the retinal pigment epithelium-choroid. n = 11–12. ** $p < 0.01$, * $p < 0.05$. From Kubota et al. [27]. Reprinted with permission. Copyright Association for Research in Vision and Ophthalmology.

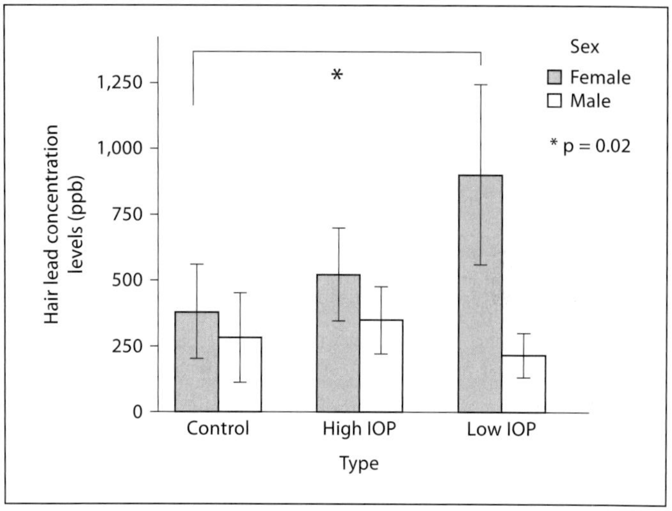

Fig. 5. Increase in lead obtained from hair in normal-tension glaucoma patients. The relation between lead accumulation in groups with high and low intraocular pressure (IOP), and control group 2. Note the significantly higher level of lead accumulation in the low-IOP group in female subjects compared to the control group in female subjects ($p = 0.02$); ppb = part per billion. From Yuki et al. [33]. Reprinted with permission from Human Press.

degeneration (AMD), photoaging might be an important mechanism in the ocular aging process. According to the free radical theory, the control of ROS can slow the aging process as well as suppress the age-related diseases.

CR and Eye Diseases

Several research studies on the effects of CR on eye disease processes have been carried out [13, 20]. Most of the data support the beneficial effect of CR on the pathology of the eye diseases. Although the concept of CR has not been applied widely to the prevention or treatment of eye diseases, we believe it has potential. Thus, we have preliminarily applied CR in the treatment of dry eye in a rat aging model. When rats age, tear volume measured by cotton thread decreases. However, when CR was applied to those aging rats by reducing the total caloric intake to 70% over 6 months, the decreased volume of tears was maintained to some extent [26].

The molecular mechanism is still unknown but this observation shed new light on the recovery of lacrimal gland dysfunction due to aging. We are now continuing this research using various animal models such as the aging mouse model. The high-fat diet model is being studied to seek the molecular changes in the lacrimal gland both in aging and CR-treated conditions.

Another approach is the use of resveratrol for the treatment of eye diseases. We performed a preliminary study on the effect of resveratrol in a lipopolysaccharide-induced uveitis model and diabetes model. Our data confirmed that resveratrol could increase the sirtuin activity in the eye (fig. 4) and suppress the inflammation in the retina [27].

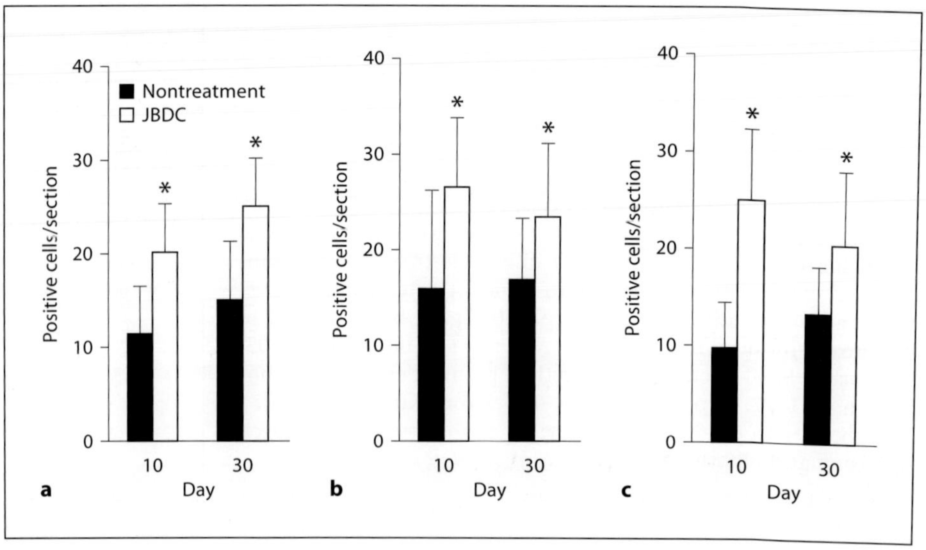

Fig. 6. Changes in oxidative stress markers in the corneal epithelia in dry eye. Note the increase in 8-hydroxy-2-deoxyguanosine (**a**), malondialdehyde (**b**) and 4-hydroxynonenal (**c**) in the cornea with the swing rat model of dry eye. Data represent the means ± SE of 16 corneas. * $p < 0.05$ versus the nontreatment group. JBDC = Swing under dry conditions. From Nakamura et al. [37]. Reprinted with permission. Copyright Association for Research in Vision and Ophthalmology.

Adhesion of the leukocyte to the vessels was also downregulated by resveratrol. Now we are applying resveratrol for the management of a dry eye animal model to assess whether it can suppress the inflammation of the lacrimal gland as well as the ocular surface. Since inflammation is considered to be a major contributing factor to the pathogenesis of dry eye, this can be a new approach for the control of dry eye in addition to cyclosporine A or other anti-inflammatory agents.

Table 1. Improvement of systemic parameters from 2001 to 2010

Parameters	2001	2006	2010
Chronological age, years	45	50	54
Biological age, years	37	33	34
Body fat, %	15.8	12.8	10.9
HbA_{1c}, %	6.1	4.7	5.1
Mercury, ppm	15.1	13.0	4.8

Data courtesy of Frontier Medical Institute, Denver, Colo., USA.

Oxidative Stress and Eye Disease

Oxidative stress and eye diseases have been well described in the literature. Especially for AMD, the large double-blind prospective Age-Related Eye Disease Study (AREDS) showed the efficacy of antioxidant supplementation to suppress the progression of AMD [28, 29], and AMD is now considered to be an oxidative stress as well as inflammatory disease. Smoking, increased body mass index, sun exposure, and accumulation of iron, lead or cadmium are the potential risk factors, suggesting also oxidative stress involvement for the pathogenesis of AMD [30–32]. Toxic heavy metals are considered to be important for the excess generation of free radicals, and a relation with the other age-related eye diseases has been found, such as increased lead levels in glaucoma patients [33] (fig. 5).

In the AREDS2 study, in addition to vitamin A, C, E and zinc and copper, lutein and zeaxanthin, eicosapentaenoic acid/docosahexaenoic acid (EPA/DHA) were the major components of the supplements [34]. Those factors are also expected to be working as antioxidants and anti-inflammatory components, but the research on the mechanism of these food factors is scarce. We have previously reported that these molecules are actually providing antioxidant and anti-inflammatory components [35, 36].

For the dry eye model, we first confirmed the accelerated oxidation of protein, fat and DNA of the ocular surface in the rat swing model (fig. 6) [37, 38]. The suppression of the blink itself can expose the ocular surface to the ambient oxygen and induce the direct oxidation of the cellular components. Then we checked whether increased free radicals could induce dry eye in the SOD1 knockout (KO) mouse. SOD is an important key enzyme for the control of O_2^-, and an increase in oxidative stress in the retina has been reported in SOD1 KO mice, induc-

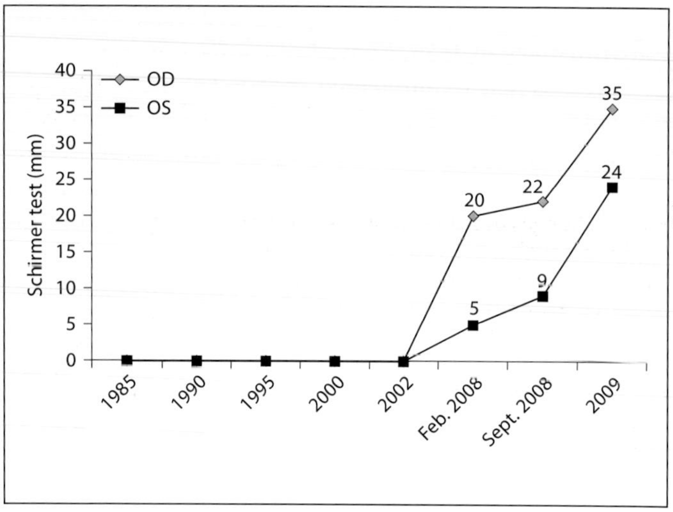

Color version available online

Fig. 7. Improvement of Schirmer test results of K.T. for over 20 years. Tear secretion shows recent increase.

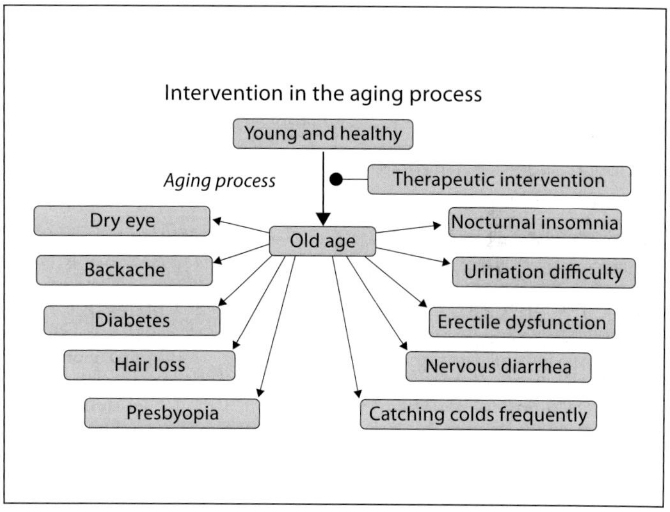

Color version available online

Fig. 8. Approach to aging itself to combat age-related conditions or diseases. Adapted from Curtis et al. [56], to my personal condition.

ing retinal aging. SOD1 KO mice clearly showed a decrease in tear volume, in addition to the compromised ocular surface. It is speculated that oxidative stress is not only involved in the deterioration of ocular surface cells, but also the dysfunction of the lacrimal gland. We are currently working on the various oxidative stress models to confirm the relationship between the ROS and dry eye.

In the clinical setting, we have shown that tobacco smoking can induce ROS in the ocular surface by initiating inflammation, resulting in dry eyes [39–41]. Since tobacco smoking is considered to be the risk factor for dry eye, it may be due to the oxidative stress. It is reported that the consumption of EPA/DHA is related to the incidence of dry eye [42], and administration of EPA might be helpful for the treatment of dry eyes. Lactoferrin is an important component in tears, which has an antioxidant effect. Our preliminary data supported that oral lactoferrin intake may increase the tear volume and ameliorate the symptoms of dry eye [43]. Other important molecules in tear fluid such as prealbumin, selenoproteins and other proteins might also be important to control the oxidative stress over the ocular surface [44–47].

Personal Experience

Although clinical research should be based on the scientific evidence such as prospective randomized intervention studies, personal experience may give rise to the opening of a new field of therapy [48]. Since the detection of dry eye during my cornea fellowship at Massachusetts Eye and Ear Infirmary in 1985, I have been suffering from severe dry eyes. When I volunteered for the Schirmer test as a normal volunteer at that time, my Schirmer test result was 0 mm in both eyes which was confirmed many times during the following year before and after I came back to Japan. Later I found that my basic tearing was 0 mm although my reflex tearing was somehow maintained. When I was diagnosed as having dry eye in 1985, I was suffering from eye discomfort but I thought it was due to the overuse of my eyes, which could be alleviated by the proper application of artificial eyedrops. This experience motivated me to establish the Dry Eye Society [49] in Japan and initiate dry eye research and education after my corneal fellowship. I have developed moisture aid glasses, autologous serum treatment and lipid application in order to decrease my dry eye condition [50–52]; however, my Schirmer test remained 0 mm in both eyes and the irritation continued.

Since many dry eye patients cannot tolerate contact lens wear due to the ocular surface desiccation, I introduced laser in situ keratomileusis (LASIK) for my patients in 1997, and to my surprise, I observed that many patients looked younger after LASIK, partially due to the wider palpebral fissure after LASIK [53]. It was during this time that I developed my interest in aging research as well as antiaging medicine. With my colleagues, we established the Japanese Antiaging Society [54] in 2001, and at the same time began the application of antiaging medicine to myself. As I have reviewed in this article, the basic idea about antiaging medicine today is CR with optimal nutrition and free radical control. I follow the basic principles of antiaging medicine by practicing CR, taking supplements and exercising, leading to the improvement of my physical parameters (table 1).

To my great surprise and joy, I noticed that my dry eye symptoms were alleviated, there was great improvement for my chronic back pain and my memory improved. The Schirmer test showed great improvement, now more than 30 mm in both eyes (fig. 7). My use of eyedrops has decreased sharply from over 50 times per day to just once or twice per day now.

Although I am still using moisture glasses during the winter in Japan and on long flights, I can avoid using them during the humid summer. Although the data from personal experience are limited to 1 subject, I am confident that dry eye can be treated in this way by applying the antiaging approach to daily practice. I hope this approach will eventually lead to the discovery of the molecular mechanism of the healing process of dry eye, leading to the development of fundamental treatment. I think we can say sometime in the near future that 'dry eye is a curable disease'.

Future Directions

The discovery of the mechanism of aging is now providing the evidence-based intervention to lifestyle, resulting in antiaging. Antiaging medicine has been a dream for many years throughout human history, but it had been just a dream without proven scientific background. Now the time has come [6, 55]. New insights into aging research have opened an interesting fundamental approach. Previously, aging diseases such as dry eye, presbyopia, back pain, diabetes and loss of hair were treated individually; however, these diseases are deeply affected by aging itself. Now the new idea of intervention in the aging process has been revealed [56]. In this model, intervention in aging can delay or possibly treat the age-related diseases. In my personal experience, many age-related conditions were solved and now I am a happy patient (fig. 8) [56].

Eye disorders such as dry eye can now be targeted by this approach. Basic as well as clinical research is under way to elucidate the mechanism. The future of antiaging medicine in ophthalmology is bright and promising.

References

1 Uchino M, Schaumberg DA, Dogru M, Uchino Y, Fukagawa K, Shimmura S, Satoh T, Takebayashi T, Tsubota K: Prevalence of dry eye disease among Japanese visual display terminal users. Ophthalmology 2008;115:1982–1988.
2 Uchino M, Dogru M, Uchino Y, Fukagawa K, Shimmura S, Takebayashi T, Schaumberg DA, Tsubota K: Japan Ministry of Health study on prevalence of dry eye disease among Japanese high school students. Am J Ophthalmol 2008;146:925–929.
3 Uchino M, Dogru M, Yagi Y, Goto E, Tomita M, Kon T, Saiki M, Matsumoto Y, Uchino Y, Yokoi N, Kinoshita S, Tsubota K: The features of dry eye disease in a Japanese elderly population. Optom Vis Sci 2006;83:797–802.
4 Xu K, Yagi Y, Tsubota K: Decrease in corneal sensitivity and changes in tear function in dry eye. Cornea 1996;15:235–239.
5 Bordone L, Guarente L: Calorie restriction, SIRT1 and metabolism: understanding longevity. Nat Rev Mol Cell Biol 2005;6:298–305.

6 Fontana L, Weiss EP, Villareal DT, Klein S, Holloszy JO: Long-term effects of calorie or protein restriction on serum IGF-1 and IGFBP-3 concentration in humans. Aging Cell 2008;7:681–687.
7 Harman D: Aging: a theory based on free radical and radiation chemistry. J Gerontol 1956;11:298–300.
8 Guarente L: Sirtuins as potential targets for metabolic syndrome. Nature 2006;444:868–874.
9 Imai S, Armstrong CM, Kaeberlein M, Guarente L: Transcriptional silencing and longevity protein Sir2 is an NAD-dependent histone deacetylase. Nature 2000;403:795–800.
10 Lee SJ, Murphy CT, Kenyon C: Glucose shortens the life span of *C. elegans* by downregulating DAF-16/FOXO activity and aquaporin gene expression. Cell Metab 2009;10:379–391.
11 Spindler SR: Calorie restriction enhances the expression of key metabolic enzymes associated with protein renewal during aging. Ann NY Acad Sci 2001;928:296–304.
12 Blagosklonny MV: An anti-aging drug today: from senescence-promoting genes to anti-aging pill. Drug Discov Today 2007;12:218–224.
13 Heilbronn LK, de Jonge L, Frisard MI, De Lany JP, Larson-Meyer DE, Rood J, et al: Effect of 6-month calorie restriction on biomarkers of longevity, metabolic adaptation, and oxidative stress in overweight individuals: a randomized controlled trial. JAMA 2006;295:1539–1548.
14 Howitz KT, Bitterman KJ, Cohen HY, Lamming DW, Lavu S, Wood JG, Zipkin RE, Chung P, Kisielewski A, Zhang LL, Scherer B, Sinclair DA: Small molecule activators of sirtuins extend *Saccharomyces cerevisiae* lifespan. Nature 2003;425:191–196.
15 Baur JA, Pearson KJ, Price NL, Jamieson HA, Lerin C, Kalra A, Prabhu VV, et al: Resveratrol improves health and survival of mice on a high-calorie diet. Nature 2006;444:337–342.
16 Pearson KJ, Baur JA, Lewis KN, Peshkin L, Price NL, Labinskyy N, et al: Resveratrol delays age-related deterioration and mimics transcriptional aspects of dietary restriction without extending life span. Cell Metab 2008;8:157–168.
17 Guarente L: Mitochondria – a nexus for aging, calorie restriction, and sirtuins? Cell 2008;132:171–176.
18 Longo VD, Kennedy BK: Sirtuins in aging and age-related disease. Cell 2006;126:257–268.
19 Matsuzawa Y: Therapy insight: adipocytokines in metabolic syndrome and related cardiovascular disease. Nat Clin Pract Cardiovasc Med 2006;3:35–42.
20 Abe T, Nakajima A, Satoh N, Ohkoshi M, Sakuragi S, Koizumi A: Suppression of experimental autoimmune uveoretinitis by dietary calorie restriction. Jpn J Ophthalmol 2001;45:46–52.
21 Obin M, Halbleib M, Lipman R, Carroll K, Taylor A, Bronson R: Calorie restriction increases light-dependent photoreceptor cell loss in the neural retina of Fischer 344 rats. Neurobiol Aging 2000;21:639–645.
22 Li Y, Wolf NS: Effects of age and long-term caloric restriction on the aqueous collecting channel in the mouse eye. J Glaucoma 1997;6:18–22.
23 Ishii N, Fujii M, Hartman PS, Tsuda M, Yasuda K, Senoo-Matsuda N, Yanase S, Ayusawa D, Suzuki K: A mutation in succinate dehydrogenase cytochrome b causes oxidative stress and ageing in nematodes. Nature 1998;394:694–697.
24 Schriner SE, Linford NJ, Martin GM, Treuting P, Ogburn CE, Emond M, Coskun PE, Ladiges W, Wolf N, Van Remmen H, Wallace DC, Rabinovitch PS: Extension of murine life span by overexpression of catalase targeted to mitochondria. Science 2005;308:1909–1911.
25 Sun J, Folk D, Bradley TJ, Tower J: Induced overexpression of mitochondrial Mn-superoxide dismutase extends the life span of adult *Drosophila melanogaster.* Genetics 2002;161:661–672.
26 Kawashima M, Kawakita T, Okada N, Ogawa Y, Murat D, Nakamura S, Nakashima H, Shimmura S, Shinmura K, Tsubota K: Calorie restriction: a new therapeutic intervention for age-related dry eye disease in rats: Biochem Biophys Res Commun 2010;397:724–728.
27 Kubota S, Kurihara T, Mochimaru H, Satofuka S, Noda K, Ozawa Y, Oike Y, Ishida S, Tsubota K: Prevention of ocular inflammation in endotoxin-induced uveitis with resveratrol by inhibiting oxidative damage and nuclear factor-kappaB activation. Invest Ophthalmol Vis Sci 2009;50:3512–3519.
28 Bressler NM, Bressler SB, Congdon NG, Ferris FL 3rd, Friedman DS, Klein R, Lindblad AS, Milton RC, Seddon JM; Age-Related Eye Disease Study Research Group: Potential public health impact of Age-Related Eye Disease Study results: AREDS report No 11. Arch Ophthalmol 2003;121:1621–1624.
29 Sackett CS, Schenning S: The Age-Related Eye Disease Study: the results of the clinical trial. Insight 2002;27:5–7.
30 Clemons TE, Milton RC, Klein R, Seddon JM, Ferris FL 3rd; Age-Related Eye Disease Study Research Group: Risk factors for the incidence of advanced age-related macular degeneration in the Age-Related Eye Disease Study (AREDS): AREDS report No 19. Ophthalmology 2005;112:533–539.
31 Erie JC, Good JA, Butz JA: Excess lead in the neural retina in age-related macular degeneration. Am J Ophthalmol 2009;148:890–894.
32 Wills NK, Kalariya N, Sadagopa Ramanujam VM, Lewis JR, Haji Abdollahi S, Husain A, van Kuijk FJ: Human retinal cadmium accumulation as a factor in the etiology of age-related macular degeneration. Exp Eye Res 2009;89:79–87.
33 Yuki K, Dogru M, Imamura Y, Kimura I, Ohtake Y, Tsubota K: Lead accumulation as possible risk factor for primary open-angle glaucoma. Biol Trace Elem Res 2009, E-pub ahead of print.
34 Coleman H, Chew E: Nutritional supplementation in age-related macular degeneration. Curr Opin Ophthalmol 2007;18:220–223.
35 Sasaki M, Ozawa Y, Kurihara T, Noda K, Imamura Y, Kobayashi S, Ishida S, Tsubota K: Neuroprotective effect of an antioxidant, lutein, during retinal inflammation. Invest Ophthalmol Vis Sci 2009;50:1433–1439.
36 Izumi-Nagai K, Nagai N, Ohgami K, Satofuka S, Ozawa Y, Tsubota K, Ohno S, Oike Y, Ishida S: Inhibition of choroidal neovascularization with an anti-inflammatory carotenoid astaxanthin. Invest Ophthalmol Vis Sci 2008;49:1679–1685.
37 Nakamura S, Shibuya M, Nakashima H, Hisamura R, Masuda N, Imagawa T, Uehara M, Tsubota K: Involvement of oxidative stress on corneal epithelial alterations in a blink-suppressed dry eye. Invest Ophthalmol Vis Sci 2007;48:1552–1558.
38 Nakamura S, Kinoshita S, Yokoi N, Ogawa Y, Shibuya M, Nakashima H, Hisamura R, Imada T, Imagawa T, Uehara M, Shibuya I, Dogru M, Ward S, Tsubota K: Lacrimal hypofunction as a new mechanism of dry eye in visual display terminal users. 2010 PLoS ONE 5:e11119.
39 Rummenie VT, Matsumoto Y, Dogru M, Wang Y, Hu Y, Ward SK, Igarashi A, Wakamatsu T, Ibrahim O, Goto E, Luyten G, Inoue H, Saito I, Shimazaki J, Tsubota K: Tear cytokine and ocular surface alterations following brief passive cigarette smoke exposure. Cytokine 2008;43:200–208.
40 Matsumoto Y, Dogru M, Goto E, Sasaki Y, Inoue H, Saito I, Shimazaki J, Tsubota K: Alterations of the tear film and ocular surface health in chronic smokers. Eye (Lond) 2008;22:961–968.
41 Altinors DD, Akça S, Akova YA, Bilezikçi B, Goto E, Dogru M, Tsubota K: Smoking associated with damage to the lipid layer of the ocular surface. Am J Ophthalmol 2006;141:1016–1021.
42 Schaumberg DA, Sullivan DA, Buring JE, Dana MR: Prevalence of dry eye syndrome among US women. Am J Ophthalmol 2003;136:318–326.
43 Dogru M, Matsumoto Y, Yamamoto Y, Goto E, Saiki M, Shimazaki J, Takebayashi T, Tsubota K: Lactoferrin in Sjögren's syndrome. Ophthalmology 2007;114:2366–2367.

44 Wakamatsu TH, Dogru M, Tsubota K: Tearful relations: oxidative stress, inflammation and eye diseases. Arq Bras Oftalmol 2008; 71(suppl):72–79.
45 Higuchi A, Shimmura S, Takeuchi T, Suematsu M, Tsubota K: Elucidation of apoptosis induced by serum deprivation in cultured conjunctival epithelial cells. Br J Ophthalmol 2006;90:760–764.
46 Higuchi A, Ueno R, Shimmura S, Suematsu M, Dogru M, Tsubota K: Albumin rescues ocular epithelial cells from cell death in dry eye. Curr Eye Res 2007;32:83–88.
47 Higuchi A, Takahashi K, Hirashima M, Kawakita T, Tsubota K: Selenoprotein p controls oxidative stress in cornea. 2010 PLoS ONE 5:e9911.
48 Todes C: Inside parkinsonism... a psychiatrist's personal experience. Lancet 1983;i: 977–978.
49 Dry Eye Society. http://www.dryeye.ne.jp.
50 Goto E, Shimazaki J, Monden Y, Takano Y, Yagi Y, Shimmura S, Tsubota K: Low-concentration homogenized castor oil eye drops for noninflamed obstructive meibomian gland dysfunction. Ophthalmology 2002; 109:2030–2035.
51 Tsubota K, Goto E, Fujita H, Ono M, Inoue H, Saito I, Shimmura S: Treatment of dry eye by autologous serum application in Sjögren's syndrome. Br J Ophthalmol 1999;83:390–395.
52 Tsubota K, Yamada M, Urayama K: Spectacle side panels and moist inserts for the treatment of dry-eye patients. Cornea 1994;13: 197–201.
53 Hori-Komai Y, Toda I, Tsubota K: Laser in situ keratomileusis: assocciation with increased width of palpebral fissure. Am J Ophthalmol 2001;131:254–255.
54 Japanese Society of Anti-Aging Medicine. http://www.anti-aging.gr.jp.
55 Colman RJ, Anderson RM, Johnson SC, Kastman EK, Kosmatka KJ, Beasley TM, Allison DB, Cruzen C, Simmons HA, Kemnitz JW, Weindruch R: Caloric restriction delays disease onset and mortality in rhesus monkeys. Science 2009;325:201–204.
56 Curtis R, Geesaman BJ, Di Stefano PS: Ageing and metabolism: drug discovery opportunities. Nat Rev Drug Discov 2005;4:569–580.

Ophthalmic Research

Ophthalmic Res 2010;44:155–165
DOI: 10.1159/000316481

Published online: September 9, 2010

Oxidative Damage and the Prevention of Age-Related Cataracts

David C. Beebe[a, b] Nancy M. Holekamp[a, c] Ying-Bo Shui[a]

Departments of [a]Ophthalmology and Visual Sciences and [b]Cell Biology and Physiology, Washington University, and [c]Barnes Retina Institute, Saint Louis, Mo., USA

Key Words
Oxidative damage · Age-related cataract

Abstract
Purpose: Cataracts are often considered to be an unavoidable consequence of aging. Oxidative damage is a major cause or consequence of cortical and nuclear cataracts, the most common types of age-related cataracts. ***Methods:*** In this review, we consider the different risk factors, natural history and etiology of each of the 3 major types of age-related cataract, as well as the potential sources of oxidative injury to the lens and the mechanisms that protect against these insults. The evidence linking different oxidative stresses to the different types of cataracts is critically evaluated. ***Results:*** We conclude from this analysis that the evidence for a causal role of oxidation is strong for nuclear, but substantially lower for cortical and posterior subcapsular cataracts. The preponderance of evidence suggests that exposure to increased levels of molecular oxygen accelerates the age-related opacification of the lens nucleus, leading to nuclear cataract. Factors in the eye that maintain low oxygen partial pressure around the lens are, therefore, important in protecting the lens from nuclear cataract. ***Conclusions:*** Maintaining or restoring the low oxygen partial pressure around that lens should decrease or prevent nuclear cataracts.

Cataracts are any opacification of the lens. Although congenital or juvenile cataracts may have serious visual consequences, early-onset cataracts contribute to a relatively small percentage of visual disability. By contrast, age-related cataracts are responsible for nearly half of all blindness worldwide and half of all visual impairment in the USA [1–3]. In the USA alone, surgery for age-related cataracts is the most expensive ocular surgical procedure, with expenditures exceeding USD 3 billion annually [4]. Lens opacities may result from protein aggregation, protein phase separation, or disturbance of the regular alignment or packing of the fiber cells, all of which may lead to increased light scattering. Nuclear opacities sometimes also involve increased coloration, resulting in decreased light transmission. Although cataracts are often considered to be an unavoidable consequence of aging, recent studies of the risk factors associated with human cataracts identified interventions that may prevent cataracts or slow their progression.

The Three Main Types of Age-Related Cataracts

Age-related lens opacities originate in 1 of 3 regions of the lens: the nucleus, cortex or the posterior pole, just beneath the posterior capsule, resulting in nuclear, cortical or posterior subcapsular cataracts (PSCs), respectively

KARGER

Fax +41 61 306 12 34
E-Mail karger@karger.ch
www.karger.com

Accessible online at:
www.karger.com/ore

Prof. David C. Beebe, PhD
Department of Ophthalmology and Visual Sciences
Washington University, Campus Box 8096
660 S. Euclid Avenue, Saint Louis, MO 63110 (USA)
E-Mail beebe@wustl.edu

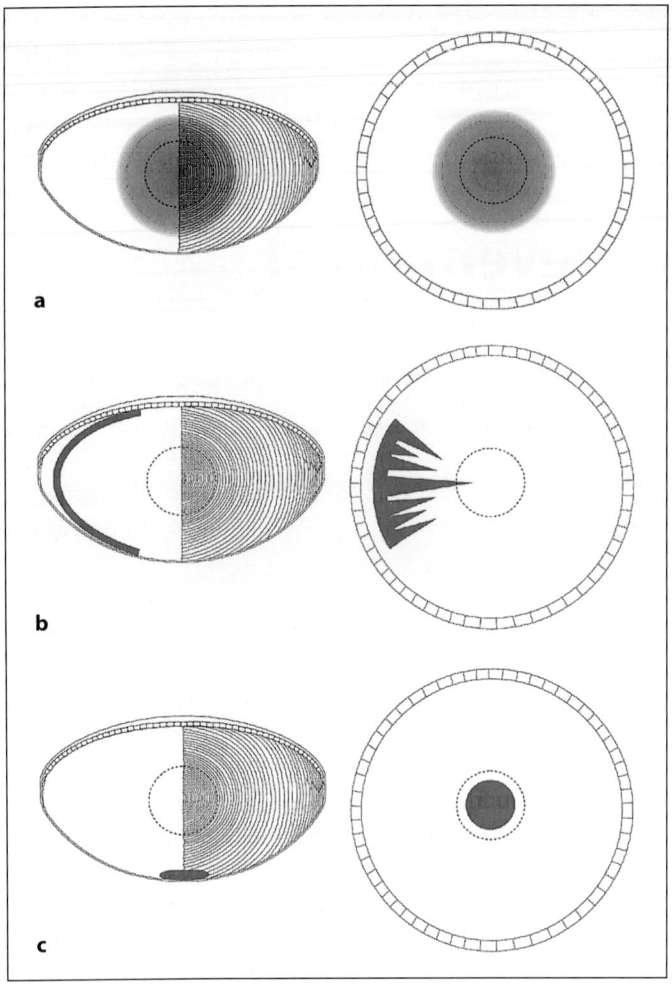

Fig. 1. Diagrams illustrating the 3 main types of age-related cataracts. **a** Nuclear cataract. A cross-sectional view of the lens is on the left. It shows the location of a nuclear opacity in the central fiber cells. The pattern of fiber cells is illustrated on the right side of this diagram. The right-hand panel in **a** shows a view of the lens, as seen through the maximally dilated pupil. The dotted circle shows the approximate location of the pupil during maximal constriction. The cataract is in the center of the visual axis. **b** Cortical cataract. An opacity in a cluster of cortical fiber cells is illustrated in cross-section on the left and as seen through the pupil on the right. Note that cortical opacities are not visually significant until the opacity reaches the visual axis. **c** PSC. A cluster of cells has accumulated at the posterior pole of the lens. The opacity is located in the visual axis, where it causes maximal degradation of visual acuity.

(fig. 1). The lens nucleus comprises approximately the central half of the lens and is composed of the fiber cells that were present at birth. Cortical opacities occur in mature (anucleate) fiber cells in the outer half of the lens, cells that were formed postnatally. PSCs form from fiber cells that fail to differentiate properly. Unlike normal fiber cells, these cells do not elongate. Instead, they migrate or are carried along with elongating fiber cells and accumulate at the posterior pole of the lens.

The prevalence of the 3 main types of age-related cataracts differs in different regions of the world and in different racial groups [5]. However, in all areas and populations, PSCs are least common. In northern Japan and northern China, cortical cataracts are more prevalent, while nuclear cataracts predominate in more southern regions of these countries [6]. Similarly, in most tropical areas, nuclear cataracts are most common. Whether these differences are related to differences in genetics, environment, diet or other factors is difficult to discern.

The 'Natural History' and Etiology of Age-Related Cataracts

Nuclear cataracts are associated with increased light scattering resulting from the aggregation and insolubilization of lens proteins and their increased association with membranes. The causes of increased aggregation are not fully understood, although increased protein oxidation is likely to be involved. During 'normal' aging, the nucleus becomes increasingly stiff, and nuclear light scattering and coloration increase. These changes are associated with increases in insoluble proteins and protein aggregation in all or nearly all persons as they age. The difference between the aging lens nucleus and the increased opacification seen in nuclear cataracts is a matter of degree. In nuclear cataracts the nucleus is substantially harder, more opaque and usually browner than in persons of similar age who are thought of as 'noncataractous'. Clinicians describe them as 'nuclear sclerotic cataracts' as an indication of the increased hardness of the cataractous nucleus.

With increasing age, many types of modifications occur in the abundant crystallin proteins of the lens nucleus. These include protein truncation, cross-linking, denaturation, amino acid racemization, deamidation, glycation and oxidation. The complexity of these changes has made it difficult to determine which might contribute to the age-related hardening and opacification of the nucleus. In contrast to these age-related changes, substantial evidence, collected over more than 50 years, implicates oxidative damage in nuclear cataracts [7].

Most of the events associated with the formation of cortical cataracts are different from those seen in nuclear cataracts. Opacification of the nucleus is not accompanied by detectable damage to the structure of nuclear fiber cells. By contrast, cortical cataracts are associated with extensive disruption of cell structure and the wholesale precipitation of intracellular proteins. Nuclear cataracts occur uniformly throughout the center of the lens, while cortical cataracts initially involve small clusters of cortical fiber cells. Unlike nuclear opacification, damage to cortical fiber cells is not a necessary consequence of aging. Most individuals never have any evidence of cortical cataracts, while everyone develops some degree of nuclear opacity with age.

The cellular disruption that occurs in cortical cataracts begins near the equator of the lens. Since cortical fiber cells extend from the posterior to the anterior of the lens, this means that opacification begins in the center of a group of fiber cells; the anterior and posterior ends of the same cells remain transparent. Morphological studies found evidence of physical damage early in cortical cataract formation, involving the scission and fragmentation of the cortical fiber cells [8, 9]. Cortical cataracts progress in severity by the involvement of increasing numbers of adjacent fiber cells and by the extension of the damage from the center of the cells to their anterior and posterior ends. Only when opacification involves the ends of the fiber cells, extending the opacity into the visual axis, does a cortical cataract impair vision.

The cellular changes that lead to the formation of PSCs have been the least studied of all types of cataracts. Examination of postmortem lenses identified streams of cells that appeared to be migrating from the equator to the posterior pole [10–12]. Microscopic examination revealed swollen cells with eosinophilic cytoplasm, suggesting fiber cells that failed to elongate. During the progression of PSCs, increasing numbers of these swollen cells accumulate along the suture planes at the posterior of the lens. Because they lie in the optic axis, these disordered clusters of cells degrade visual acuity. To our knowledge, there have been no biochemical analyses of the contents of human PSCs. Information about their etiology is limited to the risk factors associated with increased risk of developing these opacities. These are described in the following section.

Different Risk Factors for Each Type of Age-Related Cataracts

Epidemiological studies in populations from around the world identified several factors associated with an increased risk of age-related cataracts [13]. Consistent with their distinct etiologies, the risk profiles for each type of age-related cataract are also different. Based on their different risk factors and pathogenesis, we think that it is appropriate to consider each type of age-related cataract as a different disease, although they all share two common features: increasing prevalence in older individuals and opacification.

Nuclear cataracts are widely associated with poorer diet, lower socioeconomic status, nonprofessional status and lower educational achievement [2, 13]. The specific risk factors associated with these general socioeconomic categories have been difficult to discern. Clinical trials using vitamin supplementation to lower the risk of cataracts have been unsuccessful or had minimal impact, at least over the typical 5- to 10-year duration of these studies. Some supplements have potentially harmful systemic effects when used at high doses, and 1 recent study reported an increased incidence of cataract surgery in subjects taking vitamin C supplements (but not those taking multivitamin supplements or diets high in vitamin C) [14]. Smoking is a consistent risk factor for nuclear cataracts. The risk of nuclear cataracts increases with the amount and duration of smoking, adding confidence to the existence of a causal relationship between smoking and nuclear opacities. Two studies from diverse ethnic groups identified larger lens size as a risk factor for nuclear cataracts [15, 16]. Longitudinal studies showed that having a larger lens conferred increased risk of developing nuclear opacities over a 5-year follow-up period [17]. Epidemiological studies have also associated living in a region with increased ambient temperature with increased lens hardening and risk of developing nuclear cataract [6]. Although it may be difficult to establish whether higher ambient temperature is the variable responsible for the higher incidence of nuclear cataracts in these studies, recent laboratory investigations have supported this hypothesis [18]. Finally, studies of twins and examination of familial associations have suggested that about one third of the risk of nuclear cataracts is hereditary, although the genes involved have not been identified [19, 20].

High sunlight exposure has been consistently associated with an increased risk of cortical cataracts. The risk of cortical cataract attributable to sunlight is effectively eliminated by wearing a brimmed hat or plastic glasses, making sunlight exposure a preventable risk [21]. In spite of the evidence supporting a role for sunlight in cortical cataracts, the contribution of higher sunlight exposure to the total cataract burden appears to be modest. In most studies, sunlight did not contribute significantly to the risk of nuclear or posterior subcapsular opacities. Furthermore, the increased risk of cortical cataract provided by the highest levels of sunlight exposure in a typical population is only about 10% [22]. A more significant risk of developing cortical cataracts is typically associated with being female, of African heritage and having a family member with cortical cataracts [23–28]. Twin studies and family associations suggest that 50–60% of the risk of developing cortical cataracts is hereditary. The first human mutations associated with age-related cortical cataracts were recently identified in *EPH2A*, a gene encoding a transmembrane tyrosine kinase [29, 30]. It has not been determined whether it is loss of the kinase activity or the potential adhesive function of the protein that underlies these opacities. As with nuclear cataracts, lens size was identified as a significant risk factor for cortical cataracts. However, unlike nuclear cataracts, the increased prevalence and incidence of cortical opacities were linked to having a smaller, not a larger lens [15–17, 31]. Several studies have shown that diabetics also have an increased risk of developing cortical cataracts and PSCs, although diabetics with well-controlled blood sugar develop a similar spectrum of age-related cataracts as nondiabetics [32, 33].

The major risk factors associated with PSCs are high myopia, diabetes and exposure to therapeutic doses of steroids and ionizing radiation. One study, performed in rats, suggested that high-dose steroids might alter the expression of cell adhesion proteins, like E- and N-cadherin, thereby interfering with fiber cell differentiation [34]. Other than this experimental study, it remains unclear how these diverse factors lead to the defects in fiber cell differentiation that appear to underlie PSCs.

Oxidative Damage and Age-Related Cataracts

Oxidative damage is a prominent feature of nuclear and cortical cataracts. However, it is important to determine whether oxidation is the cause or the result of cataract formation.

Substantial data suggest that, with increasing age, the lens nucleus becomes more susceptible to oxidation [7]. The cytoplasm of all cells is in a 'reducing environment'. That is, oxidation is inhibited and substances that are capable of being oxidized or reduced are in the reduced state. The tripeptide glutathione is one of the most important reducing agents in the cytoplasm. Glutathione levels are extremely high in peripheral lens fiber cells, where glutathione is synthesized and reduced [35]. Reduced glutathione reaches the lens nucleus by diffusion from the surface cells through the abundant network of gap junctions in the lateral membranes of the fiber cells [36, 37]. With increasing age, a greater percentage of the glutathione in the nucleus is found in the oxidized state, as glutathione disulfide or glutathione-protein mixed disulfides. In nuclear cataracts, the proportion of glutathione that is oxidized increases further [7, 35]. In spite of this, glutathione levels in the outer cortex of the lens remain high in older lenses and in nuclear cataracts. Therefore, the increase in oxidized glutathione in the nucleus is direct evidence of local oxidation during aging and in nuclear cataracts. It also suggests that, with increasing age, the lens nucleus becomes less able to repair oxidative damage.

The factors that determine the extent of glutathione oxidation in the lens nucleus are not known with certainty. However, as the lens ages, it grows larger and its cytoplasm stiffens [38]. This means that the distance that reduced glutathione must diffuse to reach the nucleus increases, while the rate of diffusion through the lens cytoplasm decreases. At the same time, the diffusion of oxidized glutathione from the nucleus back to the lens surface, where it can be reduced, is also impaired. These changes may be sufficient to explain the increased susceptibility of the nucleus to oxidative damage in older lenses.

Cortical cataracts involve the disruption of fiber cell membranes, followed by disintegration of the cytoplasmic contents of the damaged fiber cells. Dissection of lenses with cortical cataracts releases a chalky precipitate from the cataractous areas. This is, presumably, the aggregated remains of the cytoplasmic contents. It seems possible that oxidative damage weakens or stresses the fiber cells, leading to their disruption, or that oxidation is not involved in causing cortical cataracts, but only occurs following loss of membrane integrity. Disruption of the plasma membrane would allow glutathione and other antioxidants to diffuse out of the fiber cells, resulting in the oxidation of the remaining cytoplasmic contents. For these reasons, it is difficult to decide whether cortical cataracts are caused by oxidation or whether oxidation follows the cellular disruption that precedes opacification or some of both. Answers to this conundrum may come from closer examination of the types of oxidative stress that are associated with the formation of age-related cataracts.

The Potential Causes of Oxidation in Cortical and Nuclear Cataracts

Of the risk factors identified for cortical cataracts, those that seem most likely to cause increased oxidative damage are high sunlight exposure and diabetes. It is less clear how risk factors like female sex, smaller lens size, African heritage or genetic factors might increase oxidative damage to cortical fiber cells.

Absorption of UV light can generate free radicals, leading to increased oxidative damage [39, 40]. However, there is an apparent conflict between the exposure of the eye to higher levels of UV radiation and the location of cortical cataracts. Cortical cataracts first appear at the lens equator, the region of the lens that is best protected from exposure to sunlight. This is especially true in bright light, when the pupil is maximally constricted. Similarly, the center of the lens receives the highest dose of UV radiation, yet higher sunlight exposure is not associated with nuclear cataract formation in most studies. Finally, lenses with advanced age-related nuclear color do not show evidence of UV damage, as measured by the destruction of the tryptophan residues in proteins [41]. These observations are difficult to reconcile with the concept that UV light causes cortical cataracts by directly damaging cortical lens fiber cells.

We offer two potential explanations for this paradox. UV light may be absorbed by other eye tissues, the iris, for example, which might produce toxic substances that damage cortical fiber cells [42]. This would be consistent with the increased risk of cataracts associated with dark iris color, seen in some studies [43–45]. However, in 2 of these studies, dark iris color was associated with nuclear cataracts and PSCs, not cortical cataracts.

A second possibility is that higher sunlight exposure increases the stiffness of the lens nucleus, and this increased stiffness contributes to the formation of cortical cataracts. How might this happen? As the lens ages, the nucleus becomes much stiffer, but the cortex remains soft [46]. Stiffening of the nucleus is a major contributor to presbyopia, the nearly universal inability of older individuals to focus on nearby objects [38]. Attempted accommodation by presbyopes would lead to shear forces at the boundary between the soft cortex and the stiff nucleus. If these forces damaged the membranes of cortical fiber cells, cortical cataracts might follow [9, 47].

The possibility that physical forces might underlie cortical cataracts is consistent with other risk factors. Having a smaller or thinner lens, a major risk factor for cortical cataracts, might increase the force applied to the lens during accommodation, increasing the risk of cortical damage. Among the many effects of long-term exposure to high blood sugar in diabetes is increased protein glycation, which could increase the stiffness of the nucleus, weaken the cortical fiber cells or both. The mutations in *EPH2A* that are associated with human cortical cataracts could lead to decreased strength of adhesion between fiber cells, increasing the risk of physical damage. Finally, 'mixed' nuclear and cortical cataracts are common, even though the risk factors for each type tend to be distinct. However, since nuclear cataracts are associated with hardening the nucleus, having a nuclear opacity may have the secondary effect of increasing the risk of developing a cortical cataract.

The mechanism by which diabetes damages the lens is complex and has been the subject of much debate. Persons with uncontrolled diabetes often rapidly develop cataracts. These opacities are associated with osmotic damage to the superficial lens cortex that may also involve oxidative damage [48, 49]. However, uncontrolled diabetes greatly increases mortality, making cataracts the least of the worries for these patients. As stated above, patients with well-controlled diabetes present with a spectrum of cataracts that resemble those seen in the nondiabetic population, albeit at a younger age than nondiabetics [32, 33]. This suggests that the lenses of well-controlled diabetics may be sensitized to the cataract formation, rather than diabetes being a primary cause of opacification.

Is the Lens Subjected to Especially High Levels of Oxidative Stress?

It is often stated that the lens is subjected to oxidative stress throughout life. Whether this statement is accurate or not, the absence of protein turnover and the limited ability for repair assure that any damage to the mature fiber cells will accumulate over a lifetime. Potential sources of oxidative stress to the lens include UV light, oxidants in the ocular fluids, endogenous oxidants produced in lens cells and smoke constituents.

As stated above, the connection between sunlight exposure and cortical cataracts is likely to be indirect. The iris will block light from reaching more peripheral regions of the lens and most of the shorter, more damaging wavelengths are filtered by the cornea [50]. The absorption of the UV light that does reach the lens over a lifetime does not damage the tryptophan in lens crystallins, even in cataractous lenses, suggesting that the lens is reasonably well protected from the direct effects of light. However, it has been suggested that the increase in UV-absorbing compounds in older lenses ('UV filters') may increasingly sensitize the lens to UV exposure [51]. Finally, the risk of cortical cataract that is attributable to sunlight exposure is quite small. One issue to bear in mind when weighing the epidemiological data: lifetime measures of light exposure have been based on the occupational and recreational exposure of adults. The influence of sunlight exposure in childhood has not been adequately quantified.

Potential damage to the lens from oxidants in the aqueous humor has been a controversial topic. Previous studies suggested that high levels of hydrogen peroxide are present in human aqueous humor [52]. This led to many experiments in which lenses or lens cells were exposed to hydrogen peroxide in vitro. However, the high levels of ascorbate in the aqueous humor interfere with the assay used in this initial study [53]. In addition, aqueous humor produces hydrogen peroxide when exposed to air [54]. Both considerations could lead to overestimation of the hydrogen peroxide levels in the aqueous. More recent studies, which compared the total antioxidant potential of aqueous humor from cataract and glaucoma patients, detected substantially higher antioxidant activity in the cataract patients [55]. The cataract patients also had lower levels of enzymes that are induced by exposure to oxidative stress. This observation suggests that, at least in the cataract patients included in this study, aqueous humor is unlikely to be a source of oxidative stress in cataract.

Several lines of evidence have led to the suggestion that exposure to elevated levels of molecular oxygen can cause nuclear cataracts [56–59]. However, under normal conditions, the level of oxygen around the human lens is very low, protecting the lens from this potential source of damage [58, 60]. The mechanisms that protect the lens from oxygen and the conditions under which the lens is exposed to higher levels of oxygen are discussed below.

Most cells produce endogenous oxidants as a byproduct of normal metabolism. One potential oxidant is the superoxide anion that is generated in mitochondria during oxidative phosphorylation. This potent reactive oxygen species is converted in the mitochondrion to hydrogen peroxide by superoxide dismutase. The peroxide produced may be metabolized to water by catalase activity, although the disposition of hydrogen peroxide by cells has not been carefully examined. However, lenses produce most of their ATP by glycolysis rather than oxidative phosphorylation [61]. The metabolically active cells of the lens also have very high levels of antioxidants, like glutathione. Therefore, lenses are probably less exposed to and better protected from endogenous oxidants than most other cell types.

One potential source of oxidative stress that is probably important to the lens is smoke. Smoking is one of the most reliable risk factors for nuclear cataracts in epidemiology studies throughout the world [23, 45, 62, 63]. Exposure to cooking smoke has also been linked to nuclear cataract [64]. In spite of this, we do not know which components of smoke are harmful to the lens, the mechanisms by which these components cause cataracts or even whether they directly interact with components of the lens. Given the many harmful effects of smoking, better understanding of the mechanism by which smoke causes cataracts is probably not as important as increased support for programs to reduce smoking and exposure to cooking smoke. However, understanding how smoke contributes to cataracts could be important for understanding the etiology of cataract in general.

Oxidation and Nuclear Cataracts

Clinical and experimental studies strongly implicate increased exposure of the lens to oxygen as a major cause of age-related nuclear cataracts. Patients who were treated daily for more than 1 year with hyperbaric oxygen therapy first developed a myopic shift, then incipient or full-blown nuclear cataracts [56]. A myopic shift is caused by an increase in the refractive power of the lens, presumably due to increased hardening of the lens nucleus. It is commonly a precursor to the formation of age-related nuclear (sclerotic) cataracts. Several subsequent studies of patients undergoing hyperbaric oxygen therapy confirmed the occurrence of a myopic shift, even after relatively short-term therapy [65, 66]. Importantly, these refractive changes regressed after the discontinuation of short-term therapy, suggesting that the increase in oxidation caused by hyperbaric oxygen is initially reversible. Subsequent studies in experimental animals confirmed the effect of high oxygen exposure on nuclear opacification and provided insight into some of the harmful effects of oxygen on the lens, including increased formation of protein-protein disulfide cross-links [57, 67–70]. These studies provide a direct link between excessive oxygen exposure and nuclear cataract.

Additional support for oxygen exposure in the etiology of nuclear cataracts came from studies of patients undergoing vitrectomy, the destruction and removal of the vitreous gel that is typically performed during retinal surgery. Many studies have documented very high rates of nuclear cataract formation (60–95%) within 2 years after vitrectomy surgery, and vitreoretinal surgeons counsel their patients that they will probably require cataract surgery months to a few years after vitrectomy [71–74]. As mentioned above, oxygen levels near the posterior of the human lens are very low in eyes with an intact vitreous gel (approx. 1% O_2). Oxygen levels near the lens increased markedly during vitrectomy and remained significantly elevated for months afterward [58]. Patients with ischemic diabetic retinopathy had significantly lower oxygen in their vitreous and were less likely than nondiabetics to have cataract surgery after vitrectomy [75, 76]. Our group recently completed an analysis of lens opacification following vitrectomy, using Scheimpflug photography to document the progression of nuclear opacification [Holekamp et al., Am J Ophthalmol, in press]. We found that the lenses of patients with ischemic diabetic retinopathy had lower age-adjusted nuclear opacity at baseline than those of nondiabetics and did not show a significant increase in nuclear opacification after a 1-year follow-up. By contrast, diabetics without ischemic retinopathy and nondiabetics showed rapid progression of nuclear opacity 6 and 12 months after vitrectomy. By 1 year after vitrectomy, 50% of the nonischemic patients had cataract surgery. These data are consistent with the hypothesis that vitrectomy leads to cataract formation by increasing the exposure of the lens to oxygen.

If exposure of the lens to increased oxygen can cause nuclear cataracts, it is important to understand how the low-oxygen environment around the lens is maintained in eyes that do not undergo vitrectomy. Substantial data suggest that the intact vitreous body protects against nuclear cataract and is essential to maintain the low-oxygen environment at the posterior surface of the lens. It is widely appreciated that the vitreous gel undergoes gradual collapse with age ('vitreous syneresis'). This process begins with the formation of fluid-filled lacunae near the center of the vitreous gel, which progressively coalesce. The collagen fibrils of the vitreous aggregate around the edges of these liquid-filled areas. Eventually, the collapse of the gel and the aggregation of the collagen fibrils create traction on the retina, often leading to the full or partial separation of the remaining vitreous from the retina (posterior vitreous detachment). Although the vitreous liquefies to some degree in all individuals, the extent of loss of gel vitreous can vary greatly between subjects of the same age. Postmortem studies showed that the vitreous of subjects over 50 years ranged from a nearly intact gel to one that was completely or extensively liquefied [77, 78].

Eyes with more liquefied vitreous are more likely to have nuclear opacities [78]. In subjects between 50 and 70 years old, the state of the vitreous was a better predictor of nuclear opacity than was age. Based on these data, we concluded that the intact gel vitreous preserved the low-oxygen environment around the lens by preventing mixing of the vitreous fluid (fig. 2a). In this view, oxygen diffuses into the vitreous gel from the larger retinal vessels. Microelectrode studies in animals showed that most of this oxygen is consumed by the nearby retina [79]. The consumption of oxygen by the retina maintains an oxygen gradient in the gel near the surface of the retina. However, if the gel is removed, any movements of the head or eye would result in the movement of the vitreous fluid, carrying oxygen away from the retina, mixing it with the vitreous and delivering it to the lens. In this way, the vitreous gel does not inhibit the diffusion of oxygen, but prevents its rapid distribution by fluid mixing (fig. 2b).

In addition to the protection afforded by this physical mechanism, we recently reported that the vitreous consumes oxygen [80]. Actually, it is the ascorbic acid (vitamin C) in the vitreous that reacts with oxygen, decreasing the amount of oxygen that reaches the lens. In this reaction, the ascorbate is oxidized to dehydroascorbate, which then spontaneously hydrolyzes, preventing the regeneration of ascorbate by cellular metabolism. The vitreous fluid of subjects with advanced vitreous liquefaction or previous vitrectomy had lower ascorbate and consumed oxygen more slowly than the vitreous of patients with an intact vitreous gel. The reason for the lower ascorbate and decreased oxygen consumption in eyes with no vitreous or mostly liquid vitreous is likely to be due to the increased mixing of the vitreous, which exposes more of the ascorbate to oxygen, thereby lowering ascorbate levels. Thus, the gel state of the vitreous is important to prevent the circulation of oxygen throughout the vitreous chamber and to maintain high levels of ascorbate.

The importance of the vitreous in protecting the lens from oxygen and from nuclear cataract was highlighted by studies in which the vitreous gel was intentionally preserved or destroyed. Surgery to remove preretinal membranes typically involves vitrectomy, which is soon followed by nuclear cataract. However, patients who had a variation of the usual procedure, which did not destroy the vitreous gel, did not develop nuclear cataracts, even after a 5-year follow-up [81]. These studies were important because they showed that nuclear cataract could be prevented, even in patients who had surgery to repair a

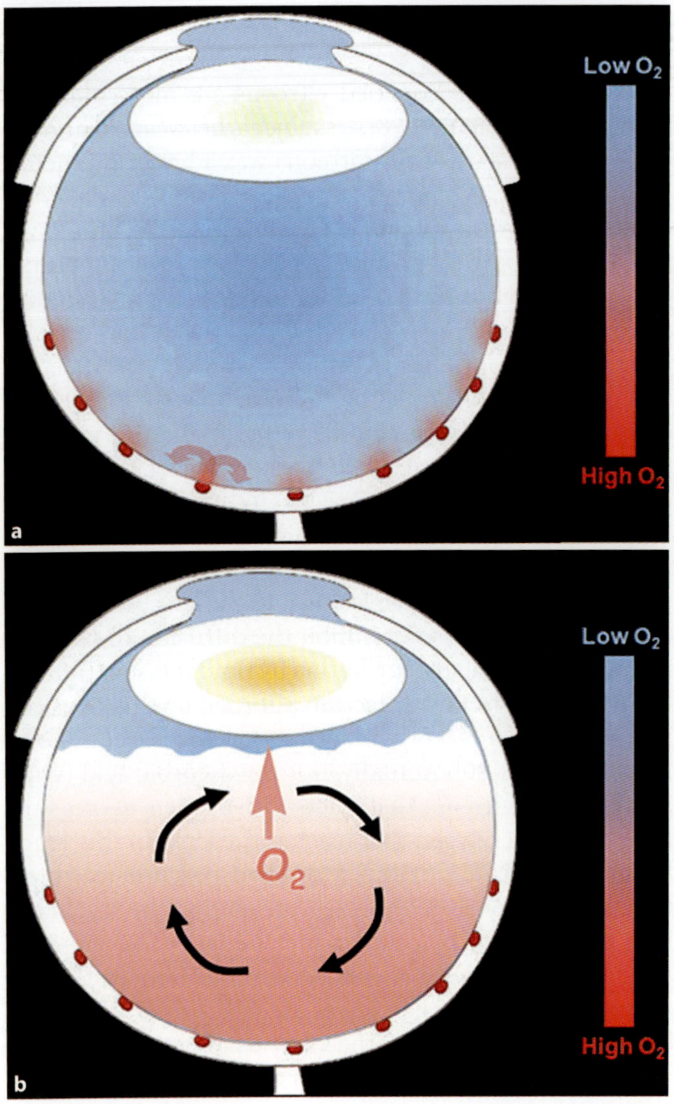

Fig. 2. Diagrams illustrating the distribution of oxygen in the normal eye and following vitrectomy or advanced vitreous degeneration. **a** An eye with an intact vitreous gel. Oxygen diffuses into the vitreous gel from the large retinal vessels. The curved arrows show that much of this oxygen is subsequently consumed by the adjacent retina. The result is a 'standing gradient' of oxygen near the retina and relatively low oxygen in the midvitreous and near the lens. The lowest oxygen partial pressure is in the midvitreous, due to the consumption of oxygen by the high concentration of ascorbic acid in the intact vitreous. **b** An eye with advanced vitreous degeneration (posterior vitreous detachment) or after vitrectomy. The posterior of the globe is filled with liquid, instead of gel. This fluid circulates when the eye moves or as a result of convection, as illustrated by the black, curved arrows. When oxygen is carried away from the retina, it can no longer be consumed by retinal metabolism. The increased mixing of oxygen with the ocular fluids delivers more oxygen to the lens (short arrow), where it leads to nuclear opacification.

retinal problem, by simply preserving the structure of the vitreous. Unfortunately, patients who had this modified procedure were more likely to have recurrence of the preretinal fibrous membranes, obviating the lens-sparing nature of the modified surgery. Recent studies in animals showed that liquefying the vitreous or creating an enzyme-induced detachment of the vitreous from the retina increased the level of oxygen in the vitreous and resulted in higher levels of oxygen reaching the lens nucleus [82, 83]. These studies demonstrate that the gel state of the vitreous protects the lens from oxygen and from nuclear cataract. The liquefaction of the vitreous, which occurs to a varying extent with age, might be considered to be a slow form of vitrectomy. Loss of the gel state of the vitreous is likely to increase the exposure of the lens to oxygen and place patients at increased risk for nuclear cataract.

Preventing Nuclear Cataract

The information described above suggests that the gel vitreous decreases the risk of nuclear cataract by protecting the lens from oxygen diffusing from the retinal vasculature. If this is correct, one might prevent nuclear cataracts by preserving the gel state of the vitreous, by replacing the vitreous gel after it is destroyed or degenerates, or by using another method to maintain a low level of oxygen around the lens.

One problem with preserving the gel state of the vitreous is that we have little information about why the vitreous liquefies with age and at a much earlier age in some individuals than in others. Without knowing the cause(s) of vitreous liquefaction, it is difficult to design interventions to preserve the vitreous gel.

Age-related changes have been detected in the fibrillar collagen network of the vitreous gel. Paul Bishop's laboratory showed that collagen IX, which coats the outer surface of the vitreous collagen fibrils, was lost at an exponentially increasing rate from human vitreous, with a half-life of 11 years [84]. Collagen IX has proteoglycan side chains that extend from the surface of the vitreous fibrils and may prevent the collapse of the collagen network. Concurrently, more of the core collagen II in the vitreous fibrils could be recognized by antibody binding. These data suggest that, with increasing age, the loss of collagen IX will lead to an increasing tendency of the fibrils of the vitreous gel to aggregate, eventually promoting the collapse of the gel. However, these changes occurred on a similar time scale in all samples, yet vitreous liquefaction occurs at quite different rates in different individuals [77, 78]. Therefore, it is possible that the degradation or modification of one or more additional components of the vitreous contributes to liquefaction.

Patients with mutations in COL2A1, COL9A1 and COL11A1 or COL11A2, the fibrillar collagens that make up the backbone of the vitreous gel, have Stickler syndrome, resulting in no or little vitreous gel from an early age (patients with mutations in COL11A1 have also been categorized as having Marshall syndrome, a related syndrome). Patients with Wagner syndrome, resulting from mutations in CSPG2, a chondroitin sulfate proteoglycan, also called versican, also have early vitreous degeneration, frequent retinal detachment and an increased risk of cataract. Early vitreous liquefaction in patients with mutations in the genes that encode these abundant components of the vitreous raises the possibility that minor variations in these genes or other structural components of the vitreous could lead to reduced stability of the vitreous gel, leading to early vitreous degeneration in some individuals. If, as suggested above, early vitreous degeneration increases the risk of nuclear cataract, variations in these genes could account for some or all of the risk of nuclear cataracts that is attributable to heredity. Since no genetic risk factors have been identified for nuclear cataracts, this possibility remains to be tested.

One of the major limitations in studying the factors that influence vitreous liquefaction is the lack of a simple, reliable, noninvasive measure of the gel state of the vitreous. Lack of such a test makes genetic and epidemiological studies of vitreous liquefaction difficult. One published method used ultrasound to quantify relatively vitreous liquefaction, but, to our knowledge, this approach has not yet been independently validated or used to screen for vitreous liquefaction [85]. If such a test were validated and easily used in the clinic, it could be used to test the association between vitreous degeneration and nuclear cataract and to identify genetic and environmental causes of vitreous liquefaction.

Several groups have developed synthetic gels to replace the vitreous after vitrectomy [86–89]. In most cases, these preparations were designed to assist in re-attaching the retina after detachment. To our knowledge, the ability of these gels to restore the low oxygen levels near the posterior surface of the lens has not been tested.

The foregoing section illustrates several opportunities to test the hypothesis that loss of the gel state of the vitreous and increased exposure of the lens to oxygen result in nuclear cataract formation. If this hypothesis were validated in human subjects, practical interventions to prevent nuclear cataracts could follow. Since vitrectomy surgery is a common procedure that causes rapid and reliable opacification of the lens nucleus, patients undergoing vitrectomy offer a promising 'model system' to test this hypothesis. Success in protecting postvitrectomy patients from developing nuclear cataracts would lay the groundwork for interventions to prevent these cataracts in subjects with advanced vitreous degeneration.

Acknowledgements

Grant funding that supported this research was provided by NIH grants EY04853 and EY15863, core grant EY02687, the BRI Research Fund and an unrestricted grant to the Department of Ophthalmology and Visual Sciences from Research to Prevent Blindness.

References

1 The Eye Diseases Prevalence Research Group: Causes and prevalence of visual impairment among adults in the United States. Arch Ophthalmol 2004;122:477–485.
2 West S: Epidemiology of cataract: accomplishments over 25 years and future directions. Ophthalmic Epidemiol 2007;14:173–178.
3 Resnikoff S, et al: Global data on visual impairment in the year 2002. Bull World Health Organ 2004;82:844–851.
4 Salm M, Belsky D, Sloan FA: Trends in cost of major eye diseases to Medicare, 1991 to 2000. Am J Ophthalmol 2006;142:976–982.
5 Sasaki K, et al: Racial differences of lens transparency properties with aging and prevalence of age-related cataract applying a WHO classification system. Ophthalmic Res 2004;36:332–340.
6 Sasaki H, et al: High prevalence of nuclear cataract in the population of tropical and subtropical areas. Dev Ophthalmol 2002;35:60–69.
7 Truscott RJW: Age-related nuclear cataract – oxidation is the key. Exp Eye Res 2004;80:709–725.
8 Brown NP, et al: Is cortical spoke cataract due to lens fibre breaks? The relationship between fibre folds, fibre breaks, waterclefts and spoke cataract. Eye 1993;7:672–679.
9 Michael R, et al: Morphology of age-related cuneiform cortical cataracts: the case for mechanical stress. Vision Res 2008;48:626–634.
10 Eshaghian J, Streeten BW: Human posterior subcapsular cataract: an ultrastructural study of the posteriorly migrating cells. Arch Ophthalmol 1980;98:134–143.
11 Eshagian J: Human posterior subcapsular cataracts. Trans Ophthalmol Soc UK 1982;102:364–368.
12 Streeten BW, Eshaghian J: Human posterior subcapsular cataract: a gross and flat preparation study. Arch Ophthalmol 1978;96:1653–1658.

13 Beebe D: Lens; in Kaufman PL, Alm A (eds): Adler's Physiology of the Eye. St Louis, Mosby, 2003, pp 117–158.
14 Rautiainen S, et al: Vitamin C supplements and the risk of age-related cataract: a population-based prospective cohort study in women. Am J Clin Nutr 2009, DOI: ajcn.2009.28528.
15 Praveen MR, et al: Lens thickness of Indian eyes: impact of isolated lens opacity, age, axial length, and influence on anterior chamber depth. Eye 2009;23:1542–1548.
16 Klein B, Klein R, Moss S: Correlates of lens thickness: the Beaver Dam Eye Study. Invest Ophthalmol Vis Sci 1998;39:1507–1510.
17 Klein BE, Klein R, Moss SE: Lens thickness and five-year cumulative incidence of cataracts: the Beaver Dam Eye Study. Ophthalmic Epidemiol 2000;7:243–248.
18 Heys KR, Friedrich MG, Truscott RJ: Presbyopia and heat: changes associated with aging of the human lens suggest a functional role for the small heat shock protein, alpha-crystallin, in maintaining lens flexibility. Aging Cell 2007;6:807–815.
19 Hammond CJ, et al: Genetic and environmental factors in age-related nuclear cataracts in monozygotic and dizygotic twins. N Engl J Med 2000;342:1786–1790.
20 Heiba IM, et al: Genetic etiology of nuclear cataract: evidence for a major gene. Am J Med Genet 1993;47:1208–1214.
21 Taylor HR, et al: Effect of ultraviolet radiation on cataract formation. N Engl J Med 1988;319:1429–1433.
22 West SK, et al: Sunlight exposure and risk of lens opacities in a population-based study: the Salisbury Eye Evaluation Project. JAMA 1998;280:714–718.
23 McCarty CA, Nanjan MB, Taylor HR: Attributable risk estimates for cataract to prioritize medical and public health action. Invest Ophthalmol Vis Sci 2000;41:3720–3725.
24 Leske MC, et al: Prevalence of lens opacities in the Barbados Eye Study. Arch Ophthalmol 1997;115:105–111.
25 Risk factors for age-related cortical, nuclear, and posterior subcapsular cataracts. The Italian-American Cataract Study Group. Am J Epidemiol 1991;133:541–553.
26 Hammond CJ, et al: The heritability of age-related cortical cataract: the Twin Eye Study. Invest Ophthalmol Vis Sci 2001;42:601–605.
27 Leske MC, Chylack LT Jr, Wu SY: The Lens Opacities Case-Control Study: risk factors for cataract. Arch Ophthalmol 1991;109:244–251.
28 Congdon N, et al: Cortical, but not posterior subcapsular, cataract shows significant familial aggregation in an older population after adjustment for possible shared environmental factors. Ophthalmology 2005;112:73–77.
29 Jun G, et al: EPHA2 is associated with age-related cortical cataract in mice and humans. PLoS Genet 2009;5:e1000584.
30 Shiels A, et al: The *EPHA2* gene is associated with cataracts linked to chromosome 1p. Mol Vis 2008;14:2042–2055.
31 Wong TY, et al: Refractive errors, axial ocular dimensions, and age-related cataracts: the Tanjong Pagar Survey. Invest Ophthalmol Vis Sci 2003;44:1479–1485.
32 Oishi N, et al: Correlation between adult diabetic cataracts and red blood cell aldose reductase levels. Invest Ophthalmol Vis Sci 2006;47:2061–2064.
33 Bron AJ, et al: The lens in diabetes. Eye 1993;7:260–275.
34 Lyu J, et al: Alteration of cadherin in dexamethasone-induced cataract organ-cultured rat lens. Invest Ophthalmol Vis Sci 2003;44:2034–2040.
35 Giblin FJ: Glutathione: a vital lens antioxidant. J Ocul Pharmacol Ther 2000;16:121–135.
36 Sweeney MHJ, Garland DL, Truscott RJW: Movement of cysteine in intact monkey lenses: the major site of entry is the germinative region. Exp Eye Res 2003;77:245–251.
37 Sweeney MH, Truscott RJ: An impediment to glutathione diffusion in older normal human lenses: a possible precondition for nuclear cataract. Exp Eye Res 1998;67:587–595.
38 McGinty SJ, Truscott RJ: Presbyopia: the first stage of nuclear cataract? Ophthalmic Res 2006;38:137–148.
39 Truscott RJW: Human cataract: the mechanisms responsible; light and butterfly eyes. Int J Biochem Cell Biol 2003;35:1500–1504.
40 Wood AM, Truscott RJ: UV filters in human lenses: tryptophan catabolism. Exp Eye Res 1993;56:317–325.
41 Harding JJ: The untenability of the sunlight hypothesis of cataractogenesis. Doc Ophthalmol 1994;88:345–349.
42 Andley UP, et al: The role of prostaglandins E_2 and $F_{2\alpha}$ in ultraviolet radiation- induced cortical cataracts in vivo. Invest Ophthalmol Vis Sci 1996;37:1539–1548.
43 Cumming RG, Mitchell P, Lim R: Iris color and cataract: the Blue Mountains Eye Study. Am J Ophthalmol 2000;130:237–238.
44 Younan C, et al: Iris color and incident cataract and cataract surgery: the Blue Mountains Eye Study. Am J Ophthalmol 2002;134:273–274.
45 AREDS: Risk factors associated with age-related nuclear and cortical cataract: a case-control study in the Age-Related Eye Disease Study, AREDS report No 5. Ophthalmology 2001;108:1400–1408.
46 Heys KR, Cram SL, Truscott RJ: Massive increase in the stiffness of the human lens nucleus with age: the basis for presbyopia? Mol Vis 2004;10:956–963.
47 Pau H: Cortical and subcapsular cataracts: significance of physical forces. Ophthalmologica 2006;220:1–5.
48 Hegde KR, Varma SD: Combination of glycemic and oxidative stress in lens: implications in augmentation of cataract formation in diabetes. Free Radic Res 2005;39:513–517.
49 Obrosova IG, Fathallah L, Lang HJ: Interaction between osmotic and oxidative stress in diabetic precataractous lens: studies with a sorbitol dehydrogenase inhibitor. Biochem Pharmacol 1999;58:1945–1954.
50 Dillon J, et al: The optical properties of the anterior segment of the eye: implications for cortical cataract. Exp Eye Res 1999;68:785–795.
51 Mizdrak J, et al: Tryptophan-derived ultraviolet filter compounds covalently bound to lens proteins are photosensitizers of oxidative damage. Free Radic Biol Med 2008;44:1108–1119.
52 Garner MH, et al: Biochemical evidence for membrane disintegration in human cataracts. Proc Natl Acad Sci USA 1981;78:1892–1895.
53 Garcia-Castineiras S, et al: Aqueous humor hydrogen peroxide analysis with dichlorophenol-indophenol. Exp Eye Res 1992;55:9–19.
54 Spector A, Ma W, Wang RR: The aqueous humor is capable of generating and degrading H_2O_2. Invest Ophthalmol Vis Sci 1998;39:1188–1197.
55 Ferreira SM, et al: Oxidative stress markers in aqueous humor of glaucoma patients. Am J Ophthalmol 2004;137:62–69.
56 Palmquist BM, Philipson B, Barr PO: Nuclear cataract and myopia during hyperbaric oxygen therapy. Br J Ophthalmol 1984;68:113–117.
57 Giblin FJ, et al: Nuclear light scattering, disulfide formation and membrane damage in lenses of older guinea pigs treated with hyperbaric oxygen. Exp Eye Res 1995;60:219–235.
58 Holekamp NM, Shui YB, Beebe DC: Vitrectomy surgery increases oxygen exposure to the lens: a possible mechanism for nuclear cataract formation. Am J Ophthalmol 2005;139:302–310.
59 Beebe DC: Maintaining transparency: a review of the developmental physiology and pathophysiology of two avascular tissues. Semin Cell Dev Biol 2008:19:125–133.
60 Helbig H, et al: Oxygen in the anterior chamber of the human eye. Ger J Ophthalmol 1993;2:161–164.
61 Winkler BS, Riley MV: Relative contributions of epithelial cells and fibers to rabbit lens ATP content and glycolysis. Invest Ophthalmol Vis Sci 1991;32:2593–2598.
62 Cumming RG, Mitchell P: Alcohol, smoking, and cataracts: the Blue Mountains Eye Study. Arch Ophthalmol 1997;115:1296–1303.
63 Hodge WG, Whitcher JP, Satariano W: Risk factors for age-related cataracts. Epidemiol Rev 1995;17:336–346.
64 Pokhrel AK, et al: Case-control study of indoor cooking smoke exposure and cataract in Nepal and India. Int J Epidemiol 2005;34:702–708.

65 Evanger K, et al: Ocular refractive changes in patients receiving hyperbaric oxygen administered by oronasal mask or hood. Acta Ophthalmol Scand 2004;82:449–453.
66 Fledelius HC, Jansen EC, Thorn J: Refractive change during hyperbaric oxygen therapy. a clinical trial including ultrasound oculometry. Acta Ophthalmol Scand 2002;80:188–190.
67 Bantseev V, et al: Effect of hyperbaric oxygen on guinea pig lens optical quality and on the refractive state of the eye. Exp Eye Res 2004; 78:925–931.
68 Gosselin MF, et al: Raman spectroscopic evidence for nuclear disulfide in isolated lenses of hyperbaric oxygen-treated guinea pigs. Exp Eye Res 2007;84:493–499.
69 Padgaonkar VA, et al: Hyperbaric oxygen in vivo accelerates the loss of cytoskeletal proteins and MIP26 in guinea pig lens nucleus. Exp Eye Res 1999;68:493–504.
70 Simpanya MF, et al: Aggregation of lens crystallins in an in vivo hyperbaric oxygen guinea pig model of nuclear cataract: dynamic light-scattering and HPLC analysis. Invest Ophthalmol Vis Sci 2005;46:4641–4651.
71 Cherfan GM, et al: Nuclear sclerotic cataract after vitrectomy for idiopathic epiretinal membranes causing macular pucker. Am J Ophthalmol 1991;111:434–438.
72 De Bustros S, et al: Nuclear sclerosis after vitrectomy for idiopathic epiretinal membranes. Am J Ophthalmol 1988;105:160–164.
73 Thompson JT, et al: Progression of nuclear sclerosis and long-term visual results of vitrectomy with transforming growth factor beta-2 for macular holes. Am J Ophthalmol 1995;119:48–54.
74 Van Effenterre G, et al: Is vitrectomy cataractogenic? Study of changes of the crystalline lens after surgery of retinal detachment. J Fr Ophtalmol 1992;15:449–454.
75 Holekamp NM, Shui Y-B, Beebe D: Lower intraocular oxygen tension in diabetic patients: possible contribution to decreased incidence of nuclear sclerotic cataract. Am J Ophthalmol 2006;141:1027–1032.
76 Smiddy WE, Feuer W: Incidence of cataract extraction after diabetic vitrectomy. Retina 2004;24:574–581.
77 O'Malley P: The pattern of vitreous syneresis: aA study of 800 autopsy eyes; inIrvine AR, O'Malley C (eds): Advances in Vitreous Surgery. Springfield, Thomas, 1976, pp 17–33.
78 Harocopos GJ, et al: Importance of vitreous liquefaction in age-related cataract. Invest Ophthalmol Vis Sci 2004;45:77–85.
79 Alder VA, Cringle SJ: Vitreal and retinal oxygenation. Graefes Arch Clin Exp Ophthalmol 1990;228:151–157.
80 Shui Y-B, et al: The gel state of the vitreous and ascorbate-dependent oxygen consumption: relationship to the etiology of nuclear cataracts. Arch Ophthalmol 2009;127:1–8.
81 Sawa M, et al: Nonvitrectomizing vitreous surgery for epiretinal membrane: long-term follow-up. Ophthalmology 2005;112:1402–1408.
82 Quiram PA, et al: Microplasmin-induced posterior vitreous detachment affects vitreous oxygen levels. Retina 2007;27:1090–1096.
83 Giblin FJ, et al: Enzyme-induced posterior vitreous detachment in the rat produces increased lens nuclear pO_2 levels. Exp Eye Res 2009;88:286–292.
84 Bishop PN, et al: Age-related changes on the surface of vitreous collagen fibrils. Invest Ophthalmol Vis Sci 2004;45:1041–1046.
85 Walton KA, et al: Age-related changes in vitreous mobility as measured by video B scan ultrasound. Exp Eye Res 2002;74:173–180.
86 Swindle-Reilly KE, et al: Rabbit study of an in situ forming hydrogel vitreous substitute. Invest Ophthalmol Vis Sci 2009;50:4840–4846.
87 Maruoka S, et al: Biocompatibility of polyvinylalcohol gel as a vitreous substitute. Curr Eye Res 2006;31:599–606.
88 Soman N, Banerjee R: Artificial vitreous replacements. Biomed Mater Eng 2003;13:59–74.
89 Suri S, Banerjee R: In vitro evaluation of in situ gels as short term vitreous substitutes. J Biomed Mater Res A 2006;79:650–664.

Ophthalmic Research

Ophthalmic Res 2010;44:166–172
DOI: 10.1159/000316477

Published online: September 9, 2010

The Importance of Nutrition in the Prevention of Ocular Disease with Special Reference to Cataract

Vaishali Agte Kirtan Tarwadi

Agharkar Research Institute, Pune, India

Key Words
Micronutrients · Antioxidants · Oxidative stress · Cataract · Ocular disease

Abstract
Background: The lens is the ocular structure most susceptible to oxidative damage. Antioxidants, micronutrients and phytochemicals have been extensively studied for their possible effects to prevent or delay the progression of various eye diseases. ***Objectives:*** A brief overview of the updated literature on the role of antioxidants and micronutrients in the prevention and treatment of ocular diseases is to be presented with an emphasis on cataract. ***Data Sources:*** PubMed search and individual papers from journals. ***Data Synthesis:*** The review discusses linkages of various micronutrients and antioxidants as well as oxidative stress with cataract. Dietary interventions as strategy for prevention of cataract and other ocular disorders are also reviewed. ***Conclusions:*** Consumption of food-based antioxidants like β-carotene lutein and zeaxanthin seem to be useful for the treatment of macular degeneration and cataracts. Supplements of vitamin A, vitamin C, vitamin E and zinc may prevent advanced age-related macular degeneration only in high-risk individuals.

Introduction

Ocular diseases such as cataracts, glaucoma and age-related macular degeneration (AMD) are common causes of blindness, which is the second biggest fear, next to death, among the elderly. Cataract formation represents a serious problem in the elderly and has a large impact on the health care budget. The lens is the ocular structure most susceptible to oxidative damage. In addition to cellular death and degeneration, when the underlying epithelial cells are exposed to the action of exogenous and endogenous reactive oxygen species, the crystallin proteins in the lens cross-link and aggregate, resulting in cataracts. Oxidative stress is a crucial factor in age-related processes including cataract formation. The form and intensity of oxidative stress determine the cataract type and pigmentation, making efforts in the cataract prevention challenge more complex. Disturbance of balance between oxidative processes and antioxidative defenses causes the oxidative stress that can damage proteins, lipids, polysaccharides and nucleic acids of the ocular tissues. Among other factors, obesity, smoking, aging and diabetes accelerate degenerative processes. Their numerous consequences that appear in the eye are well known. However, inadequate antioxidant statuses being a crucial determi-

KARGER

Fax +41 61 306 12 34
E-Mail karger@karger.ch
www.karger.com

0030–3747/10/0443–0166$26.00/0

Accessible online at:
www.karger.com/ore

Dr. Vaishali Vilas Agte
Agharkar Research Institute
G.G. Agharkar Road
Pune 411 004 (India)
Tel. +91 20 2565 4357, Fax +91 20 2565 1542, E-Mail vaishaliagte@hotmail.com

nant, antioxidant micronutrients and phytochemicals have been extensively studied for their possible effects to prevent or delay the progression of various eye diseases. Food-based antioxidant nutrients might be useful in the treatment of macular degeneration and cataracts. This paper presents a brief overview of the updated literature of these explorations with an emphasis on cataract.

Nutrition and Cataract

Linkages of Macronutrients, Micronutrients and Antioxidants with Cataract

There have been numerous studies in different populations for examining the associations of micronutrients and antioxidants with cataract. In a study on levels of vitamin C, vitamin E, glutathione and lipopolysaccharide for 42 cataract patients and 40 age-matched controls, persons with cataract had lower levels of vitamin C and higher levels of vitamin B_6 and selenium [1]. Glutathione has been proven to be a potent antioxidant, and its deficiency has been implicated in cataractogenesis [2].

The nutritional deprivation or an insult to the lens protein before or soon after birth may trigger cataractogenesis [3, 4] as seen in the cohort study in a population of 1,428 English men and women aged 64–74 years, in which the body weight at 1 year was negatively correlated with the nuclear opacity score in adult life ($p = 0.001$). The association remained after controlling for age, sex, smoking, social class, adult height and diabetes.

To evaluate associations with biochemical indicators of nutritional and other risk factors for cataractogenesis, Leske et al. [5], conducted the Lens Opacities Case-Control Study on 1,380 participants (40–79 years). Odds ratios were significantly decreased for glycine (0.36) and aspartic acid (0.31). Lens opacities were associated with lower levels of riboflavin, vitamin E, iron and protein nutritional status. Higher levels of uric acid were associated with increased risk of mixed opacities. Vitamins of the B group and other antioxidant vitamins and cataract risk were also investigated [6]: a negative association between β-carotene and vitamin E intakes and relative risk of cataract implicated that development of lens opacities can be prevented by antioxidant micronutrients.

A number of studies have shown a decreased cataract risk in people with high plasma levels of antioxidant micronutrients (vitamins A, C and E) [7–10]. However, the findings of a protective effect are not consistent, and the interpretation of these findings remains limited by the wide variety of methods used and parameters measured. Selenite cataract was due to an oxidative stress to the lens, where ascorbate functioned as an anticataractogenic substance [11]. Dietary and supplemental intakes of antioxidant micronutrients were monitored prospectively for 4 years in women with intact lenses recruited from the Nurses' Health Study (n = 50,828; 45–67 years). After 8 years, the incidence of cataract extraction was lower in women with high antioxidant scores [12]. Additionally, the consumption of a vitamin C supplement for more than 10 years conferred a significant, 45% reduction in the risk of developing cataract.

The studies on Indians revealed that inadequacies of certain micronutrients, such as riboflavin, zinc and copper, were associated with cataract [13, 14]. In undernourished patients, the proportion of insoluble proteins in the lens was found to be significantly higher as compared to well-nourished cataract patients, indicating a decreased solubility of soluble proteins, a common finding in nuclear cataracts [15]. Previous work carried out by our group indicated compromised plasma levels of ascorbic acid, β-carotene, riboflavin, thiamine, zinc and selenium in 140 senile cataract patients as compared to 100 age- and sex-matched controls [16]. A protective effect of antioxidants on lens tissue and supplementation with vitamin C and lutein/zeaxanthin have been associated with a decreased risk of cataract formation in multiple observational studies. However, in a review of the carotenoids lutein and zeaxanthin, the US Food and Drug Administration has concluded that there is insufficient evidence to suggest that supplementation with these carotenoids lowers the risk of cataract formation but these nutrients may help individuals exposed to high oxidative stress, such as heavy smokers, and those with poor nutrition [17].

Oxidative Stress and Cataract

In cataract, the lens being the main target tissue, oxidative stress as a result of increased generation of active species of oxygen and free radicals in the lens have been implicated in the etiology/pathogenesis of age-related cataract resulting in loss of transparency, degeneration of biochemical parameters such as ATP, GPD, nonprotein thiols, and oxidation of lens protein and lipid [18, 19]. Among environmental factors, UVB radiation [20] and cigarette smoke are important oxidants in the pathogenesis of cataract. Lipopolysaccharide formation could be one of the mechanisms of cataractogenesis [21].

To understand the biochemical and molecular mechanisms underlying lens browning and cataractogenesis, a wide range of biochemical parameters were investigated in human cataracts. An increased aggregation and cross-linking, conformational change, crystallin susceptibility to UVB (290–320 nm) radiation, denaturation and protein oxidation accompanied by reduced glutathione, ascorbic acid and protein sulfhydryl groups, and decrease in enzymatic antioxidant defense as observed by catalase and glutathione peroxidase in the cortical region during lens browning and cataract formation have been reported [22].

Oxidative as well as osmotic stress caused by accumulation of polyols within the lens has been shown to be associated with glucose-induced cataractogenesis. Taurine has an antioxidant capacity, and its level in diabetic cataractous lens is markedly decreased. An in vitro lens culture study has indicated that taurine might spare glutathione and protect the lens from oxidative stress induced by a high concentration of glucose [23].

Effect of Supplementation of Selected Micronutrients

Considering the reported significant associations of micronutrient deficiencies with cataract, some prospective studies on supplementation have been conducted but gave controversial results. In the Age-Related Eye Disease Study (AREDS) [24] on 111 senile cataract patients, a high-dose formulation of vitamin C, vitamin E and β-carotene in a relatively well-nourished cohort had no apparent effect on the progression of age-related lens opacities. However, another study on participants from the same cohort (n = 247 women; 56–71 years) in support of vitamin C supplementation (400–700 mg daily) for at least 10 years was associated with a 77% lower prevalence of early lens opacities and an 83% lower prevalence of moderate lens opacities.

In 1 more longitudinal study of cataract, changes in nuclear opacification were measured over 5 years in 764 participants older than 40 years [25]. The risk of progression of nuclear cataracts was reduced by one third and one half in subjects who regularly consumed a multivitamin or vitamin E supplements, respectively, as well as in those with higher plasma levels of vitamin E. Contrary to these findings, however, an end-of-trial random sample of 1,828 middle-aged male smokers in the Finnish ATBC study (α-tocopherol, β-carotene cancer prevention study) showed no effect on cataract prevalence after 5–8 years of supplementation with these nutrients [26].

Further support of a protective effect against developing age-related cataracts, by antioxidant micronutrients and/or vitamin/mineral supplements, has been derived from the 2 landmark cataract intervention trials in Linxian, China, by Sperduto et al. [27], when participants over 65 years who took the supplements had a 36% lower prevalence of nuclear cataract. In the general population trial, prevalence of nuclear cataract was significantly lower in those who received a riboflavin/niacin, retinol/zinc and the vitamin C/molybdenum supplements [27].

To determine if a mixture of oral antioxidant micronutrients, i.e. β-carotene (18 mg/day), vitamin C (750 mg/day) and vitamin E (600 mg/day), would modify progression of age-related cataract, a multicentered, prospective, double-masked, randomized, placebo-controlled, 3-year trial was undertaken by Chylack et al. [28] using serial digital retroillumination imagery of the lens when there was a small positive treatment effect in US patients ($p = 0.0001$); after 3 years, a positive effect was apparent ($p = 0.048$) in both the US and the UK groups.

Trace Elements in Cataractous Lens

A number of studies have reported the concentration of inorganic elements (zinc, copper, iron, calcium, potassium, sodium, selenium and manganese) in the cataractous lens [29–32] when an increase was found for zinc, copper and calcium; the potassium was the same as compared with the normal lenses, and no significant changes were seen for selenium values. To investigate the possible influence of diabetes on the zinc and iron content of the lens, iron and zinc of 57 human lenses (28 corticonuclear cataracts and 29 capsular cataracts) were analyzed by Dawczynski et al. [33]. Diabetic patients had both increased zinc and iron contents in the lens compared to nondiabetic subjects especially for the advanced forms of cataract and dark brown colored lenses of diabetics. Our data also support this observation when the trace metal profiles of lenses between diabetic and nondiabetic cataract patients were compared [34].

Levels of zinc (11 mg/l) and copper (0.8 mg/l) were determined by Sethi et al. [35] and Srivastava et al. [36] in the nucleus of the lens of Indian cataract patients. The results showed that copper and zinc content increased, although more in the cortex than nucleus sections of the cataractous lens. Concentrations of lead, zinc, potassium, calcium, copper and sodium were determined in several human cataract and clear lenses, obtained from patients from 2 contrasting environmental regions from Delhi, India [37], in which it was observed that the intrusion of lead and calcium ions and extrusion of zinc and potassium ions through the process of ion exchange occurred in the cataractous lens, thereby influencing its transparency.

Effects of Multiple Micronutrient Supplements

One thousand twenty participants, 55–75 years old and with early or no cataract, were randomly assigned to a daily tablet of a multivitamin/mineral formulation or a placebo. Lens events were less common in participants who took the multivitamin/mineral formulation, but the treatment had opposite effects on the development or progression of nuclear and posterior subcapsular cataract opacities [38]. To examine the relation between dietary intake of carotenoids and vitamins C and E and the risk of cataract in women, the diet of 35,551 women without cataract provided detailed information on antioxidant nutrient intake from food and supplements. Higher dietary intakes of lutein/zeaxanthin and vitamin E from food and supplements were associated with significantly decreased risks of cataract [39].

The summary of the role of nutritional factors in lens opacity is shown in figure 1.

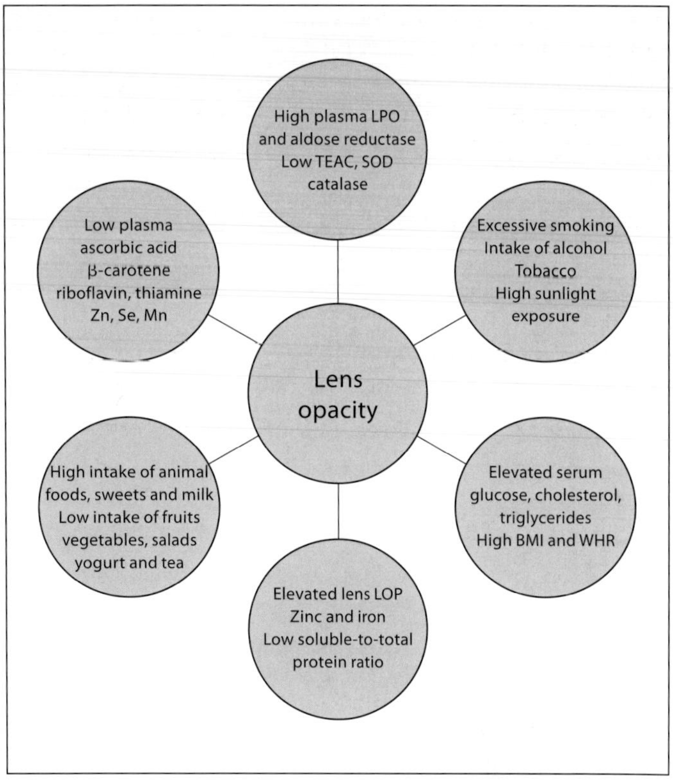

Fig. 1. Linkages of dietary, nutritional and lifestyle factors with lens opacity. LPO = Lipopolysaccharide; TEAC = Trolox equivalent antioxidant capacity; SCD = superoxide dismutase; BMI = body mass index; WHR = waist-hip ratio.

Dietary Interventions as Strategy for Prevention of Other Ocular Disorders

As with cardiovascular disease, nutrition and environmental intervention present new clinical practice and research opportunities in eye care. This includes maximizing health potential with food choice, the use of supplementation in high-risk and noncompliant patients, avoiding toxins such as cigarettes, and encouraging exercise. Lutein and zeaxanthin, two xanthophylls that have been considered to delay formation of eye diseases (AMD, cataract), are found in numerous dietary supplements advised for eye protection or supply of nutritional components [40].

The role of nutritional supplementation is of increasing interest with regard to ocular disease. Randomized controlled trials have demonstrated the effectiveness of supplementation for AMD, and formulations are now being developed for use by people with diabetes and diabetic retinopathy. Medline and Embase searches were based on 50 trials which identified a positive effect of chromium on fasting plasma glucose. Isoflavones were found to have a positive effect on insulin resistance and cardiovascular outcome measures, but only when combined with soy proteins. Vitamin E is reported to reduce oxidative stress at levels of 200 mg/day or more [41]. The field of micronutrients is currently being developed in ophthalmology. As observed in cardiovascular diseases, AMD, ocular surface diseases and even glaucoma could benefit from dietary modifications. Among the different fundamental dietary elements, the role of lipids and essential fatty acids seems particularly interesting [42]. Published studies and information found in PubMed, International Bibliographic Information of dietary supplements and selected websites have been reviewed by West et al. [43] for the role of nutritional and herbal medicines in the treatment of AMD, cataract, diabetic retinopathy and glaucoma. The available evidence does support the use of certain vitamins and minerals in patients with certain forms of AMD. For cataracts, the available evidence does not support these supplements to prevent or treat cataracts in healthy individuals. For diabetic retinopathy and glaucoma, the available evidence does not support the use of these supplements. In the category of herbal medicines, the available evidence does not support the use of herbal medicines for any of these ocular diseases.

The role of nutritional supplementation in the prevention of onset or progression of ocular disease is of interest to health care professionals and patients. Literature searches were carried out on Web of Science and PubMed

Table 1. Nutrients for ocular health

Nutrient/antioxidant	Role in vision	Rich sources	Health impacts
Vitamin E	Potent free radical scavenger	Sunflower seeds, almonds, hazelnuts	Prevention of cataracts and AMD
Vitamin A	night blindness, dry eyes	Cod liver oil, beef and chicken liver, carrots, kale	Prevention of blindness and cataracts, improves vision
β-Carotene	Precursor of vitamin A	Green leafy vegetables	Prevention of cataracts
Lutein and zeaxanthin	Powerful free radical scavengers, protect the retina	Green and yellow vegetables and egg yolks	Prevention of cataracts and retinopathy
Lycopene	Potent free radical scavenger	Red tomatoes	Prevention of cataracts
Zinc	Helps in absorption of vitamin A, acts as cofactor for superoxide dismutase	Oysters, hamburgers, wheat and nuts	Prevention of cataracts and AMD, improves immune functioning
Selenium	Helps in absorption of vitamin E, constituent of glutathione peroxidase	Brazil nuts, yeast and seafood like oysters	Prevention of cataracts and AMD
Quercetin	Strong phenolic antioxidant and free radical scavenger, antiallergic, anti-inflammatory, anticarcinogenic, antiviral and antithrombotic properties	Onions, capers, cranberries, fennel, cocoa, black currants, buckwheat, black tea	Prevention of cataracts and AMD
L-Carnitine	Protects the neurons of the optic nerve, protects vision	Red beef, artichokes, asparagus, beet greens, broccoli, garlic, mustard greens, okra and parsley	Prevention of cataracts and AMD, strengthens the immune system

for articles relating to the use of nutrients in ocular disease such as vitamins A, B, C and E, carotenoids β-carotene, lutein and zeaxanthin, minerals selenium and zinc, and the herb *Ginkgo biloba*. It has been advocated that vitamins C and E, and lutein/zeaxanthin should be included in our theoretically ideal ocular nutritional supplement [44]. However, nutritional supplements are not without risks, and their effects must be diligently and accurately monitored. However, they pose a potentially useful complement for treating ocular disease and conditions [45]. Table 1 lists the nutrients that play an important role in maintaining vision.

Role of Oxidative Stress in Other Ocular Disorders

Oxidative stress is a term used to describe any challenge in which pro-oxidants predominate over antioxidants; it may be due to either increased production of reactive oxygen species or decreased levels of antioxidants (enzymatic and nonenzymatic) or both.

Primary open-angle glaucoma (POAG) is a complex chronic neurological disease that can result in blindness. Although epidemiological studies of POAG have not addressed the role of nutrition in the development of POAG, some papers have considered that nutrition may have an impact on POAG patients. The pathway for elastin remodeling and apoptosis induction seems to be influenced by endogenous lipid-soluble antioxidants, for example vitamin E. Roles can be defined for antioxidants in the two different pathways of extracellular matrix remodeling and apoptosis induction [46].

Linkages of Micronutrient Status with Prevalence of Ocular Disorders

Among the large sample size studies, e.g. in the Beaver Dam Eye Study, the association of use of vitamin, mineral and nonvitamin nonmineral supplements with common age-related eye diseases has been investigated in 13,985 participants. There was little evidence of any significant associations between supplement use and incident ocular outcomes except for a small protective effect for cortical cataracts by vitamins A and D, zinc and multivitamins as well as increased odds of late AMD. Late AMD was associated with incident use of vitamins A, C and E and zinc. AMD seems to precede the use of vitamins A, C and E and zinc. This may reflect advice by family, friends and health care providers about the benefits of supplements similar to those in the AREDS [47].

Among several theories involved in the pathogenesis of POAG, the vascular theory considers the disease to be a consequence of reduced ocular blood flow associated with red blood cell abnormalities. Linear regressions predicted that red blood cell choline plasmalogen levels would decrease years before clinical symptoms, whereas the levels of phosphatidyl choline carrying docosahexaenoic acid were linearly correlated with visual field loss. These data demonstrate the selective loss of some individual phospholipid species in red blood cell membranes, which may partly explain their loss of flexibility in POAG [48].

Conclusions

Understanding about the importance of micronutrients in the control and prevention of ocular diseases has been relatively recent. There appear to be significant health benefits from dietary antioxidants from fruits and vegetables, in particular β-carotene, lutein and zeaxanthin, for the treatment of macular degeneration and cataracts. Epidemiological studies on cataract have suggested that antioxidant micronutrients such as α-tocopherol, retinol and ascorbic acid may help to protect against cataractogenesis. However, there are conflicting results in this area. Further, supplements of vitamin A, vitamin C, vitamin E and zinc may prevent advanced AMD only in high-risk individuals.

References

1 Jacques PF, Hartz SC, Chylack LT Jr, McGandy RB, Sadowski JA: Nutritional status in persons with and without senile cataract: blood vitamin and mineral levels. Am J Clin Nutr 1988;48:152–158.

2 Giblin FJ: Glutathione: a vital lens antioxidant. J Ocul Pharmacol Ther 2000;16:121–135.

3 Rauf A, Evans JR, Wormald RP: Relation of fetal and infant growth to adult eye disease. I. Lens opacities. Invest Ophthalmol Vis Sci 1996;37:S237.

4 Evans JR, Rauf A, Sayer AA: Age-related nuclear lens opacities are associated with reduced growth before 1 year of age. Invest Ophthalmol Vis Sci 1998;39:1740–1744.

5 Leske MC, Wu SY, Hyman L, Sperduto R, Underwood B, Chylack LT, Milton RC, Srivastava S, Ansari N: Biochemical factors in the lens opacities: case-control study. The Lens Opacities Case-Control Study Group. Arch Ophthalmol 1995;113:1113–1119.

6 Jacques PF, Hartz SC, Chylack LT Jr, McGandy RB, Sadowski JA: Nutritional status in persons with and without senile cataract: blood vitamin and mineral levels. Am J Clin Nutr 1988;48:152–158.

7 Jacques PF, Taylor A, Hankinson SE: Long-term vitamin C supplements and prevalence of early age-related lens opacities. Am J Clin Nutr 1997;66:911–916.

8 Knekt P, Jarvinen R, Seppanen R, Heliovaara M, Teppo L, Aroma A: Dietary flavonoids and the risk of lung cancer and other malignant neoplasms. Am J Epidemiol 1997;146:223–230.

9 Casado A, Torre R, Lopez-Fernandez E: Antioxidant enzyme levels in red blood cells from cataract patients. Gerontology 2001;47:186–188.

10 Cumming RG, Mitchell P, Smith W: Diet and cataract. The Blue Mountains Eye Study. Ophthalmology 2000;107:450–456.

11 Devamanoharan PS, Henein M, Morris S, Ramachandran S, Richards RD, Varma SD: Prevention of selenite cataract by vitamin C. Exp Eye Res 1991;52:563–568.

12 Hankinson SE, Stampfer MJ, Seddon JM: Nutrient intake and cataract extraction in women: a prospective study. Br Med J 1992;305:335–339.

13 Bhat KS: Plasma tryptophan levels in subjects with mature cataract. Afro-Asian J Ophthalmol 1988;7:89–90.

14 Rao PV, Bhat KS: Influence of dietary riboflavin deficiency on lenticular glutathione redox cycle, lipid peroxidation and free radical scavengers in the rat. J Clin Biochem Nutr 1989;6:195–204.

15 Bhat KS: Alterations in the lenticular proteins of rats on riboflavin deficient diet. Curr Eye Res 1983;2:829–834.

16 Tarwadi KV, Agte VV: Potential of commonly consumed green leafy vegetables for their antioxidant capacity and their linkage with micronutrient profile. Int J Food Sci Nutr 2003;56:417–425.

17 Fernandez MM, Afshari NA: Nutrition and the prevention of cataracts. Curr Opin Ophthalmol 2008;19:66–70.

18 Taylor A, Nowell T: Oxidative stress and antioxidant function in relation to risk for cataract. Adv Pharmacol 1997;38:515–536.

19 Shansi F, Sharkey E, Creighton D, Nagaraj R: Maillard reactions in lens proteins: methylglyoxal mediated modifications in rat lens. Exp Eye Res 2000;70:369–380.

20 Balasubramanian D: Ultraviolet radiation and cataract. J Ocul Pharm Ther 2000;16:285–297.

21 Donma O, Yorulmaz E, Pekel H, Syugul N: Blood and lens lipid peroxidation and antioxidant status in normal individuals, senile and diabetic cataractous patients. Curr Eye Res 2002;25:9–16.

22 Bhat KS: Scavengers of peroxide and related oxidants in human brunescent cataracts; in Gupta SK (ed): Ocular Pharmacology: Recent Advances. New Delhi, India, Indian Ocular Pharmacological Society, 1991, pp 32–38.

23 Sun J, Chu YF: Antioxidant and antiproliferative activities of common fruits. J Agric Food Chem 2002;50:7449–7454.

24 Age-Related Eye Disease Study Research Group: A randomized, placebo-controlled, clinical trial of high-dose supplementation with vitamins C and E and beta-carotene for age-related cataract and vision loss. AREDS report No 9. Arch Ophthalmol 2001;119:1439–1452.

25 Leske MC, Wu SY, Hyman L, Sperduto R, Underwood B, Chylack LT, Milton RC, Srivastava S, Ansari N: Biochemical factors in the lens opacities: case-control study. The Lens Opacities Case-Control Study Group. Arch Ophthalmol 1995;113:1113–1119.

26 Teikari JM, Virtamo J, Rautalahti M: Long-term supplementation with alpha-tocopherol and beta-carotene and age-related cataract. Acta Ophthalmol Scand 1997;75:634–640.

27 Sperduto RD, Hu T-S, Milton RC: The Linxian Cataract Studies: two nutrition intervention trials. Arch Ophthalmol 1993;111:1246–1253.

28 Chylack LT Jr, Brown NP, Bron A, Hurst M, Kopcke W, Thien U, Schalch W: The Roche European American Cataract Trial (REACT): a randomized clinical trial to investigate the efficacy of an oral antioxidant micronutrient mixture to slow progression of age-related cataract. Ophthalmic Epidemiol 2002;9:49–80.

29 Swanson A, Truesdale A: Elemental analysis in normal and cataract human lens tissue. Biochem Biophys Res Commun 1971;45:1488–1496.

30 Rasi V, Costantini S, Moramarco A, Giordano R, Giustolisi R, Balacco Gabrieli C: Inorganic element concentrations in cataractous human lenses. Ann Ophthalmol 1992;24:459–464.

31 Stanojevic-Paovic A, Hristic V, Cuperlovic M, Jovanovic S, Krsmanovic J: Macro- and microelements in the cataractous eye lens. Ophthalmic Res 1987;19:230–234.

32 Chen CZ: Analysis of 7 elements in the serum and lens of senile cataract patients. Zhonghua Yan Ke Za Zhi 1992;28:355–357.

33 Dawczynski J, Blum M, Winnefeld K, Strobel J: Increased content of zinc and iron in human cataractous lenses. Biol Trace Elem Res 2002;90:15–23.

34 Agte V, Tarwadi K: Combination of diabetes and cataract worsens the oxidative stress and micronutrient status in Indians. Nutrition 2008;24:617–624.

35 Sethi A, Nath K, Ahmed N: Trace elements and cataracts: a comparative study of trace element levels in patients with mature senile cataracts. Proceedings of the International Symposium on Trace Elements, Paris, France, 1987, pp 151–153.

36 Srivastava VK, Varshney N, Pandey DC: Role of trace elements in senile cataract. Acta Ophthalmol 1992;70:839–841.

37 Shukla N, Moitra JK, Trivedi RC: Determination of lead, zinc, potassium, calcium, copper and sodium in human cataract lenses. Sci Total Environ 1996;181:161–165.

38 Maraini G, Williams SL, Camparini M, Baratta G, Lamedica A, et al: A randomized, double-masked, placebo-controlled clinical trial of multivitamin supplementation for age-related lens opacities. Clinical trial of nutritional supplements and age-related cataract report No 3. Ophthalmology 2008;115:599–607.

39 Christen WG, Liu S, Glynn RJ, Gaziano JM, Buring JE: Dietary carotenoids, vitamins C and E, and risk of cataract in women: a prospective study. Arch Ophthalmol 2008;126:1606–1607.

40 Hamułka J, Nogal D: The assessment and characteristic of dietary supplements with lutein and zeaxanthin on the Polish pharmaceutical market. Rocz Panstw Zakl Hig 2008;59:47–57.

41 Bartlett HE, Eperjesi F: Nutritional supplementation for type 2 diabetes: a systematic review. Ophthalmic Physiol Opt 2008;28:503–523.

42 Creuzot-Garcher C, Bron A: The place of micronutrition in glaucoma management. J Fr Ophtalmol 2008;31:2S65–68.

43 West AL, Oren GA, Moroi SE: Evidence for the use of nutritional supplements and herbal medicines in common eye diseases. Am J Ophthalmol 2006;141:157–166.

44 Bartlett H, Eperjesi F: An ideal ocular nutritional supplement? Ophthalmic Physiol Opt 2004;24:339–349.

45 Blodi BA: Nutritional supplements in the prevention of age-related macular degeneration. Insight 2004;29:15–16.

46 Veach J: Functional dichotomy: glutathione and vitamin E in homeostasis relevant to primary open-angle glaucoma. Br J Nutr 2004;91:809–829.

47 Klein BE, Knudtson MD, Lee KE, Reinke JO, Danforth LG, Wealti AM, Moore E, Klein R: Supplements and age-related eye conditions: the Beaver Dam Eye Study. Ophthalmology 2008;115:1203–1208.

48 Acar N, Berdeaux O, Juaneda P, Grégoire S, Cabaret S, Joffre C, Creuzot-Garcher CP, Bretillon L, Bron AM: Red blood cell plasmalogens and docosahexaenoic acid are independently reduced in primary open-angle glaucoma. Exp Eye Res 2009;89:840–853.

Ophthalmic Research

Ophthalmic Res 2010;44:173–178
DOI: 10.1159/000316478

Published online: September 9, 2010

Mechanisms of Retinal Ganglion Cell Injury in Aging and Glaucoma

Vicki Chrysostomou Ian A. Trounce Jonathan G. Crowston

Centre for Eye Research Australia, Department of Ophthalmology, University of Melbourne, Royal Victorian Eye and Ear Hospital, East Melbourne, Vic., Australia

Key Words
Aging · Ganglion cell injury · Glaucoma

Abstract
Aging is the greatest risk factor for glaucoma, implying that intrinsic age-related changes to retinal ganglion cells, their supporting tissue or both make retinal ganglion cells susceptible to injury. Changes to the ocular vasculature, connective tissue of the optic nerve head and mitochondria, which have been documented with advancing age and shown to be exacerbated in glaucoma, may predispose to glaucomatous injury. When considering such age-related changes, it is difficult to separate pathological change from physiological change, and cause from consequence. The insults that predispose aged retinal ganglion cells to injury are likely to be varied and multiple; therefore, it may be more relevant to identify and treat common mechanisms that predispose to retinal ganglion cell failure and/or death. We suggest that mitochondrial dysfunction, as either a cause or consequence of injury, renders retinal ganglion cells sensitive to degeneration. Therapeutic approaches that target mitochondria and promote energy production may provide a general means of protecting aged retinal ganglion cells from degeneration, regardless of the etiology.

Introduction

Glaucoma is an optic neuropathy characterized by the accelerated death of retinal ganglion cells and their axons. The prevalence of glaucoma increases markedly with advancing age (fig. 1) across all populations [1, 2]. While glaucoma has traditionally been considered a disease of raised intraocular pressure (IOP), the increase in disease prevalence with age is not accompanied by a corresponding increase in IOP [3]. Furthermore, not all ocular hypertensive patients develop glaucoma, not all glaucoma patients have elevated IOP, and lowering IOP does not always prevent vision loss in glaucoma patients. These observations imply that age-associated changes, which are independent of IOP, make retinal ganglion cells more vulnerable to degeneration.

An increase in the susceptibility of aged retinal ganglion cells to injury has been demonstrated in a number of experimental models. Retinal ganglion cells suffer greater damage in response to optic nerve crush or ischemia-reperfusion in old compared to young rodents [4–6]. Age-related susceptibility to degeneration is seen in other regions of the central nervous system; aging is the greatest risk factor for Parkinson's disease, Alzheimer's disease and amyotrophic lateral sclerosis [7]. However, the pathophysiology that predisposes aging neurons to

KARGER

Fax +41 61 306 12 34
E-Mail karger@karger.ch
www.karger.com

0030–3747/10/0443–0173$26.00/0

Accessible online at:
www.karger.com/ore

Jonathan G. Crowston
Glaucoma Research Unit, Centre for Eye Research Australia
Royal Victorian Eye and Ear Hospital, 32 Gisborne Street
East Melbourne, Vic. 3002 (Australia)
Tel. +61 3 9929 8429, Fax +61 3 9662 3859, E-Mail crowston@unimelb.edu.au

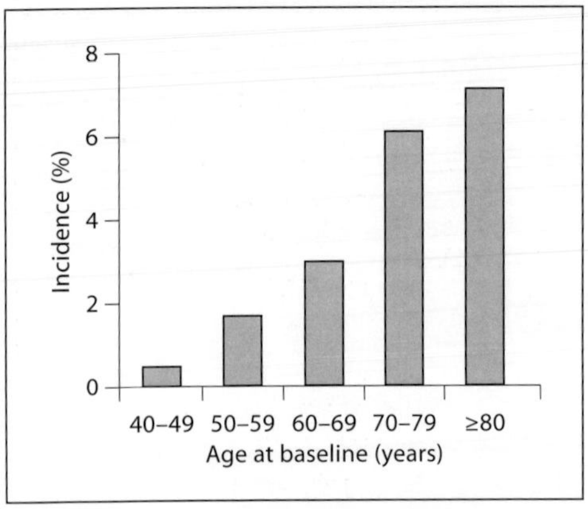

Fig. 1. Five-year age-specific incidence of glaucoma. The overall incidence of open-angle glaucoma increases near-exponentially with advancing age. Data adapted from the population-based Melbourne Visual Impairment Project [2].

degeneration remains unclear. Here, we will consider some key changes to retinal ganglion cells and their microenvironment that are seen in aging and exacerbated in glaucoma. We will also consider the mechanisms by which these changes may contribute to glaucomatous degeneration and the interaction between them.

Mechanisms of Retinal Ganglion Cell Injury

Vascular Insufficiency

Vascular insufficiency can be caused by vasospastic events that impair autoregulation, hemodynamic changes that reduce perfusion pressure such as hypotension and changes to vessel walls, or hematological changes that increase vascular resistance such as an increase in blood viscosity. Regardless of the underlying cause, vascular insufficiency results in compromised oxygen supply, nutrient delivery and waste removal.

In Aging

Structural changes to the ocular vasculature are seen with increasing age and include basement membrane thickening, increased vessel tortuosity, loss of capillary patency, vessel kinking and narrowing of arterioles and venules [8, 9]. Changes to ocular vascular dynamics including blood flow, volume and velocity with advancing age have been reported in the ophthalmic artery [10, 11], central retinal artery [12], in capillaries of the neuroretinal rim [13, 14], lamina cribrosa [14, 15] and optic nerve head [16] and also in the choroid [17, 18]. Age-related changes are not always evident with some studies reporting no correlation between age and ocular blood flow [19, 20]. These discrepancies may relate to different measurement techniques and patient populations. Overwhelmingly, however, the current body of literature supports a reduction in ocular blood flow with age.

In Glaucoma

Retinal ganglion cells are some of the most metabolically active cells in the body, making them particularly sensitive to any circulatory abnormalities that decrease oxygen and nutrient supply. As such, vascular insufficiency and the associated ischemic insult to retinal ganglion cells are implicated in the pathogenesis of glaucoma. It has been shown that primary open-angle glaucoma (POAG) patients have an impaired blood flow in the central retinal artery [21–23], inner retinal vasculature [24], optic nerve head [25, 26], ophthalmic artery [27, 28] and choroid [29, 30]. Collectively, these findings support a role for vascular insufficiency in glaucoma although caution must be taken in interpreting the results due to heterogeneous patient groups, small group sizes, differing measurement techniques, the unknown effect of antiglaucoma medications and the varying comparison of POAG patients with either healthy or ocular hypertensive patients. Systemic hypotension [31] and other systemic hematological defects such as increased plasma viscosity [24] and hypercoagulation [32] have also been reported in glaucoma patients and may exacerbate or contribute to disturbances in ocular blood flow.

Mechanical Damage

The lamina cribrosa of the optic nerve head is a series of perforated connective tissue plates through which blood vessels and retinal ganglion cell axons pass. The extracellular matrix of the lamina cribrosa is composed of various types of collagen, elastin, proteoglycans and glycoproteins, presumably synthesized by astrocytes located on the surface of the plates. Structural remodeling of the lamina cribrosa is thought to cause misalignment of connective tissue plates, resulting in compressive forces that act on directly underlying vessels and axons. This is likely to result in reduced diffusion of nutrients and oxygen from laminar capillaries to retinal ganglion cell axons.

In Aging

Significant structural change is seen in the lamina cribrosa with advancing age. Increased laminar beam thickness [33, 34], increased astrocyte basement membrane thickness [35, 36], hardening of the extracellular matrix [33, 37], increased collagen and elastin content [33, 38] and changes to proteoglycans and glycosaminoglycans [39] are seen when old tissue is compared to young tissue. In combination or alone, these age-related changes make the aged optic nerve head significantly stiffer and less compliant than the young optic nerve head.

In Glaucoma

Because damage to retinal ganglion cells within the lamina cribrosa is a central pathology of glaucoma, much research has focused on optic nerve head remodeling in the glaucomatous eye. Predictions of how alterations in optic nerve head structure underlie the clinical behavior and increased susceptibility of the aged optic nerve to glaucomatous damage have been presented recently by Burgoyne and Downs [40].

In animal models, changes to the prelaminar, laminar and peripapillary scleral tissues of the optic nerve head have been described at the earliest detectable stages of experimental glaucoma. These changes include displacement, thickening and hardening of the lamina cribrosa [41, 42], deformation of the neural canal [43] and alteration of collagen and elastin fibers in the extracellular matrix of the lamina cribrosa [44, 45]. Many of these studies were performed using young animals in which IOP was experimentally elevated, indicating that IOP alone can cause the aforementioned changes to optic nerve head tissues. Alterations to the lamina cribrosa in human glaucomatous eyes have also been reported, including changes in the types of collagen fibers [46, 47], abnormal biosynthesis of elastin [48] and thickening of basement membranes [45, 48].

Mitochondrial Dysfunction

Mitochondria are central to cell survival and integrity. In addition to providing cellular energy via oxidative phosphorylation, mitochondria regulate several key processes such as apoptosis, cell growth, calcium homeostasis and production of reactive oxygen species (ROS). Mitochondria are particularly susceptible to damage due to a close proximity to ROS production and a lack of DNA protection by histones.

In Aging

It is well accepted that mitochondria accumulate structural and functional damage with age. Although studies specifically looking at the retina and optic nerve are lacking, age-associated mitochondrial dysfunction has been described in a range of other human tissues including the central nervous system [7]. Changes to mitochondria that are seen with advancing age include increased mitochondrial DNA (mtDNA) mutations, a reduction in mitochondrial mass, reduced rates and efficiency of oxidative phosphorylation and increased production of ROS.

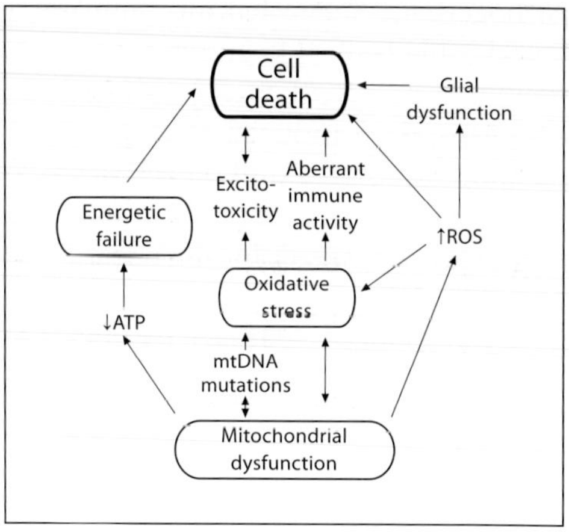

Fig. 2. Potential pathways through which mitochondrial dysfunction can lead to retinal ganglion cell death.

In Glaucoma

Due to their high rates of metabolism, retinal ganglion cells contain high numbers of mitochondria that are concentrated along unmyelinated axons. Retinal ganglion cells are specifically sensitive to mitochondrial abnormalities, as evidenced by the optic neuropathies Leber's hereditary optic neuropathy and autosomal dominant optic atrophy, both of which are caused by mitochondrion-related genetic defects and both of which result in the selective loss of retinal ganglion cells. An association between mitochondrial dysfunction and glaucoma has recently been shown in a clinical study reporting increased mtDNA mutations and a reduction in mitochondrial respiratory function in the peripheral blood of POAG patients compared to age-matched controls [49]. In a similar way, somatic mtDNA mutations are seen in association with age-related neurodegenerative conditions such as Parkinson's disease, Alzheimer's disease, amyotrophic lateral sclerosis and age-related hearing loss [7].

An immediate consequence of mitochondrial dysfunction is decreased ATP synthesis and increased production of ROS due to leakage through the electron transport chain (fig. 2). There is a large body of literature implicating ROS and associated oxidative stress in glaucoma pathogenesis. Suggested mechanisms include direct cytotoxic effects of ROS on retinal ganglion cells, ROS signaling as a second messenger in retinal ganglion cell apoptosis, ROS-induced glial dysfunction as a cause for secondary retinal ganglion cell death, oxidative damage as an activator of aberrant immune responses or oxidative stress as a trigger for the release of excitotoxic amino acids [50, 51].

While oxidative damage by ROS is often considered a cause for cell degeneration in glaucoma and other neurodegenerative diseases, the energetic failure associated with mitochondrial dysfunction may be more relevant. We hypothesize that age-related mitochondrial dysfunction renders retinal ganglion cells susceptible to glaucomatous injury by reducing the energy available for repair processes and predisposing cells to apoptosis. This idea has recently been reviewed in more detail by us [52] and others [53].

Interactions

Above, we have outlined 3 age-related changes to retinal ganglion cells and their supporting tissues that may predispose cells to glaucomatous degeneration. Many other changes to ocular tissue have been described with advancing age and may also be involved in the pathogenesis of glaucoma. Some of these changes include condensation of the vitreous gel, alteration of corneal tonicity and scleral rigidity, changes to the shape and tone of the ciliary body, decreased lumen area of the aqueous collecting channel, changes in the width of the anterior chamber, decreased rates of optic nerve axonal transport, deterioration of the blood-retina barrier and increased numbers of microglia and activated immune cells.

Importantly, the interaction between various age-related changes and the concepts of cause versus consequence, and pathological change versus physiological change, must be considered. For example, vascular insufficiency may arise as a secondary consequence of structural changes to the lamina cribrosa and optic nerve head. Alternatively, if glaucoma is a primary vascular disease, circulatory disturbances may lead to remodeling of the lamina cribrosa. A reduction in nutrient and oxygen supply caused by, or as a consequence of, structural changes to the lamina cribrosa may affect the efficiency of mitochondrial respiration in the prelaminar region.

It must be realized that increasing age does not independently give rise to disease. More likely, aging, via a number of changes, generates increasingly vulnerable vasculature, connective tissue and retinal ganglion cells that are susceptible to subsequent insult. The rate and extent of insult will be further influenced by genes and environment that determine the rate of aging in every individual.

Methods of Protecting Retinal Ganglion Cells from Injury

Given the cause for retinal ganglion cell damage in glaucoma is likely to be multifactorial, general neuroprotective treatments that increase the resistance of retinal ganglion cells to injury may have the most successful outcomes. We believe therapies that target mitochondria and enhance energy production in retinal ganglion cells will provide this protection, a concept also proposed by Osborne [53]. The importance of mitochondria in mediating cell survival is clear. One of the most widely employed methods of slowing the aging process and delaying the onset of age-related disease is calorie restriction. Resveratrol, a mimetic of calorie restriction, has also gained much attention recently. Both calorie restriction and resveratrol have been shown to protect against neurodegeneration, and early reports indicate that this protection extends to the retina [5, 54, 55]. There is strong evidence that the benefits of these interventions are mediated by mitochondria. Both calorie restriction and resveratrol induce mitochondrial biogenesis, the formation of new mitochondria within cells, and improve mitochondrial function [56]. Another means of enhancing mitochondrial function is exercise. Physical activity is a potent stimulator of mitochondrial biogenesis in muscle, heart and brain, which leads to enhanced oxidative phosphorylation activity and a corresponding increase in oxygen consumption and ATP synthesis [57–59]. Although the modulating effects of exercise on retinal mitochondria are yet to be shown, preliminary evidence suggests that vigorous physical activity may reduce glaucoma risk [60]. Mitochondrion-targeted therapies for protecting retinal ganglion cells from injury represent an exciting avenue of future research.

Conclusion

Changes in ocular vasculature, the supporting tissue of the optic nerve head and retinal ganglion cell mitochondria with advancing age may all predispose to glaucomatous optic neuropathy. Strong associations between these age-related changes and glaucoma have been described. When considering age-related changes that are relevant to retinal ganglion cell loss in glaucoma, it is important to distinguish physiological from pathological changes, and primary from secondary effects. It is unlikely that any single event will explain retinal ganglion cell injury in all forms of glaucoma or that the underlying cause for injury is the same in every individual. It is more likely that the collection of changes associated with increasing age leads to an increasingly vulnerable optic nerve. We postulate that interventions aimed at delaying or reversing these age-related changes, for example by promoting mitochondrial biogenesis, may restore the ability of retinal ganglion cells to respond to injury of any type, thus improving disease outcomes in glaucoma.

Acknowledgements

Centre for Eye Research Australia receives Operational Infrastructure Support from the Victorian Government.

References

1 Quigley HA, Broman AT: The number of people with glaucoma worldwide in 2010 and 2020. Br J Ophthalmol 2006;90:262–267.
2 Dimitrov PN, et al: Five-year incidence of bilateral cause-specific visual impairment in the Melbourne Visual Impairment Project. Invest Ophthalmol Vis Sci 2003;44:5075–5081.
3 Varma R, et al: Prevalence of open-angle glaucoma and ocular hypertension in Latinos: the Los Angeles Latino Eye Study. Ophthalmology 2004;111:1439–1448.
4 Katano H, et al: Effects of aging on the electroretinogram during ischemia-reperfusion in rats. Jpn J Physiol 2001;51:89–97.
5 Kim K-Y, Ju W-K, Neufeld AH: Neuronal susceptibility to damage: comparison of the retinas of young, old and old/caloric restricted rats before and after transient ischemia. Neurobiol Aging 2004;25:491–500.
6 Wang AI, Yuan M, Neufeld AH: Age-related changes in neuronal susceptibility to damage. Ann NY Acad Sci 2007;1097:64–66.
7 Lin MT, Beal MF: Mitochondrial dysfunction and oxidative stress in neurodegenerative diseases. Nature 2006;443:787–795.
8 Hughes S, et al: Altered pericyte-endothelial relations in the rat retina during aging: implications for vessel stability. Neurobiol Aging 2006;27:1838–1847.
9 Leung H, et al: Relationships between age, blood pressure, and retinal vessel diameters in an older population. Invest Ophthalmol Vis Sci 2003;44:2900–2904.
10 Lam AK, et al: The effect of age on ocular blood supply determined by pulsatile ocular blood flow and color Doppler ultrasonography. Optom Vis Sci 2003;80:305–311.
11 Ravalico G, et al: Age-related ocular blood flow changes. Invest Ophthalmol Vis Sci 1996;37:2645–2650.
12 Groh MJ, et al: Influence of age on retinal and optic nerve head blood circulation. Ophthalmology 1996;103:529–534.
13 Boehm AG, Koeller AU, Pillunat LE: The effect of age on optic nerve head blood flow. Invest Ophthalmol Vis Sci 2005;46:1291–1295.
14 Embleton SJ, et al: Effect of senescence on ocular blood flow in the retina, neuroretinal rim and lamina cribrosa, using scanning laser Doppler flowmetry. Eye (Lond) 2002;16:156–162.
15 Nicolela MT, et al: Ocular hypertension and primary open-angle glaucoma: a comparative study of their retrobulbar blood flow velocity. J Glaucoma 1996;5:308–310.
16 Rizzo JF 3rd, et al: Optic nerve head blood speed as a function of age in normal human subjects. Invest Ophthalmol Vis Sci 1991;32:3263–3272.
17 Grunwald JE, Hariprasad SM, Du Pont J: Effect of aging on foveolar choroidal circulation. Arch Ophthalmol 1998;116:150–154.
18 Ito YN, et al: Aging changes of the choroidal dye filling pattern in indocyanine green angiography of normal subjects. Retina 2001;21:237–242.
19 Harris A, et al: Aging affects the retrobulbar circulation differently in women and men. Arch Ophthalmol 2000;118:1076–1080.
20 Williamson TH, Lowe GD, Baxter GM: Influence of age, systemic blood pressure, smoking, and blood viscosity on orbital blood velocities. Br J Ophthalmol 1995;79:17–22.
21 Bergstrand IC, et al: Timolol increased retrobulbar flow velocities in untreated glaucoma eyes but not in ocular hypertension. Acta Ophthalmol Scand 2001;79:455–461.
22 Kaiser HJ, et al: Blood-flow velocities of the extraocular vessels in patients with high-tension and normal-tension primary open-angle glaucoma. Am J Ophthalmol 1997;123:320–327.
23 Yamazaki Y, Drance SM: The relationship between progression of visual field defects and retrobulbar circulation in patients with glaucoma. Am J Ophthalmol 1997;124:287–295.
24 Wolf S, et al: Retinal hemodynamics using scanning laser ophthalmoscopy and hemorheology in chronic open-angle glaucoma. Ophthalmology 1993;100:1561–1566.
25 Kerr J, Nelson P, O'Brien C: A comparison of ocular blood flow in untreated primary open-angle glaucoma and ocular hypertension. Am J Ophthalmol 1998;126:42–51.
26 Michelson G: Perfusion of the juxtapapillary retina and the neuroretinal rim area in primary open angle glaucoma. J Glaucoma 1996;5:91–98.
27 Arend O, et al: Pathogenetic aspects of the glaucomatous optic neuropathy: fluorescein angiographic findings in patients with primary open angle glaucoma. Brain Res Bull 2004;62:517–524.
28 Rojanapongpun P, Drance SM, Morrison BJ: Ophthalmic artery flow velocity in glaucomatous and normal subjects. Br J Ophthalmol 1993;77:25–29.
29 Kerr J, Nelson P, O'Brien C: Pulsatile ocular blood flow in primary open-angle glaucoma and ocular hypertension. Am J Ophthalmol 2003;136:1106–1113.
30 Trew DR, Smith SE: Postural studies in pulsatile ocular blood flow. II. Chronic open angle glaucoma. Br J Ophthalmol 1991;75:71–75.
31 Collignon N, et al: Ambulatory blood pressure monitoring in glaucoma patients: the nocturnal systolic dip and its relationship with disease progression. Int Ophthalmol 1998;22:19–25.
32 O'Brien C, et al: Activation of the coagulation cascade in untreated primary open-angle glaucoma. Ophthalmology 1997;104:725–729.
33 Albon J, et al: Age related compliance of the lamina cribrosa in human eyes. Br J Ophthalmol 2000;84:318–323.
34 Kotecha A, Izadi S, Jeffery G: Age-related changes in the thickness of the human lamina cribrosa. Br J Ophthalmol 2006;90:1531–1534.
35 Hernandez MR, Luo XX, Andrzejewska W: Age-related changes in the extracellular matrix of the human optic nerve head. Am J Ophthalmol 1989;107:476–484.

36 Hernandez MR, et al: Localization of collagen types I and IV mRNAs in human optic nerve head by in situ hybridization. Invest Ophthalmol Vis Sci 1991;32:2169–2177.
37 Morrison JC, et al: Aging changes of the rhesus monkey optic nerve. Invest Ophthalmol Vis Sci 1990;31:1623–1627.
38 Morrison JC, et al: Structural proteins of the neonatal and adult lamina cribrosa. Arch Ophthalmol 1989;107:1220–1224.
39 Albon J, et al: Age related changes in the non-collagenous components of the extracellular matrix of the human lamina cribrosa. Br J Ophthalmol 2000;84:311–317.
40 Burgoyne CF, Downs JC: Premise and prediction: how optic nerve head biomechanics underlies the susceptibility and clinical behavior of the aged optic nerve head. J Glaucoma 2008;17:318–328.
41 Yang H, et al: 3-D histomorphometry of the normal and early glaucomatous monkey optic nerve head: lamina cribrosa and peripapillary scleral position and thickness. Invest Ophthalmol Vis Sci 2007;48:4597–4607.
42 Burgoyne CF, et al: Three-dimensional reconstruction of normal and early glaucoma monkey optic nerve head connective tissues. Invest Ophthalmol Vis Sci 2004;45:4388–4399.
43 Downs JC, et al: Three-dimensional histomorphometry of the normal and early glaucomatous monkey optic nerve head: neural canal and subarachnoid space architecture. Invest Ophthalmol Vis Sci 2007;48:3195–3208.
44 Johnson EC, et al: The effect of chronically elevated intraocular pressure on the rat optic nerve head extracellular matrix. Exp Eye Res 1996;62:663–674.
45 Quigley HA, Brown A, Dorman-Pease ME: Alterations in elastin of the optic nerve head in human and experimental glaucoma. Br J Ophthalmol 1991;75:552–557.
46 Hernandez MR, Ye H, Roy S: Collagen type IV gene expression in human optic nerve heads with primary open angle glaucoma. Exp Eye Res 1994;59:41–52.
47 Tengroth B, Ammitzboll T: Changes in the content and composition of collagen in the glaucomatous eye – basis for a new hypothesis for the genesis of chronic open angle glaucoma – a preliminary report. Acta Opthalmol 1984;62:999–1008.
48 Hernandez MR: Ultrastructural immunocytochemical analysis of elastin in the human lamina cribrosa: changes in elastic fibers in primary open-angle glaucoma. Invest Ophthalmol Vis Sci 1992;33:2891–2903.
49 Abu-Amero KK, Morales J, Bosley TM: Mitochondrial abnormalities in patients with primary open-angle glaucoma. Invest Ophthalmol Vis Sci 2006;47:2533–2541.
50 Izzotti A, Bagnis A, Saccà SC: The role of oxidative stress in glaucoma. Mutat Res 2006; 612:105–114.
51 Tezel G: Oxidative stress in glaucomatous neurodegeneration: mechanisms and consequences. Prog Retin Eye Res 2006;25:490–513.
52 Kong GYX, et al: Mitochondrial dysfunction and glaucoma. J Glaucoma 2009;18:93–100.
53 Osborne NN: Pathogenesis of ganglion 'cell death' in glaucoma and neuroprotection: focus on ganglion cell axonal mitochondria. Prog Brain Res 2008;173:339–352.
54 Kubota S, et al: Prevention of ocular inflammation in endotoxin-induced uveitis with resveratrol by inhibiting oxidative damage and nuclear factor-κB activation. Invest Ophthalmol Vis Sci 2009;50:3512–3519.
55 Liu Q, et al: Oxidative stress is an early event in hydrostatic pressure induced retinal ganglion cell damage. Invest Ophthalmol Vis Sci 2007;48:4580–4589.
56 Lopez-Lluch G, et al: Calorie restriction induces mitochondrial biogenesis and bioenergetic efficiency. Proc Natl Acad Sci USA 2006;103:1768–1773.
57 Boveris A, Navarro A: Systemic and mitochondrial adaptive responses to moderate exercise in rodents. Free Radic Biol Med 2008;44:224–229.
58 Dietrich MO, Andrews ZB, Horvath TL: Exercise-induced synaptogenesis in the hippocampus is dependent on UCP2-regulated mitochondrial adaptation. J Neurosci 2008; 28:10766–10771.
59 Holloszy JO: Regulation by exercise of skeletal muscle content of mitochondria and GLUT4. J Physiol Pharmacol 2008;59(suppl 7):5–18.
60 Williams PT: Relationship of incident glaucoma versus physical activity and fitness in male runners. Med Sci Sports Exerc 2009;41: 1566–1572.

Ophthalmic Research

Ophthalmic Res 2010;44:179–190
DOI: 10.1159/000316480

Published online: September 9, 2010

The Importance of Mitochondria in Age-Related and Inherited Eye Disorders

Stuart G. Jarrett[a] Alfred S. Lewin[b] Michael E. Boulton[c]

[a]Department of Molecular and Biomedical Pharmacology, College of Medicine, University of Kentucky, Lexington, Ky., [b]Department of Molecular Genetics, University of Florida, and [c]Department of Anatomy and Cell Biology, College of Medicine, University of Florida, Gainesville, Fla., USA

Key Words

Mitochondria · Ocular function · Reactive oxygen species

Abstract

Mitochondria are critical for ocular function as they represent the major source of a cell's supply of energy and play an important role in cell differentiation and survival. Mitochondrial dysfunction can occur as a result of inherited mitochondrial mutations (e.g. Leber's hereditary optic neuropathy and chronic progressive external ophthalmoplegia) or stochastic oxidative damage which leads to cumulative mitochondrial damage and is an important factor in age-related disorders (e.g. age-related macular degeneration, cataract and diabetic retinopathy). Mitochondrial DNA (mtDNA) instability is an important factor in mitochondrial impairment culminating in age-related changes and pathology, and in all regions of the eye mtDNA damage is increased as a consequence of aging and age-related disease. It is now apparent that the mitochondrial genome is a weak link in the defenses of ocular cells since it is susceptible to oxidative damage and it lacks some of the systems that protect the nuclear genome, such as nucleotide excision repair. Accumulation of mitochondrial mutations leads to cellular dysfunction and increased susceptibility to adverse events which contribute to the pathogenesis of numerous sporadic and chronic disorders in the eye.

Introduction

Accumulating evidence supports a role for mitochondrial dysfunction in aging and disease in a wide range of tissues resulting in sporadic and chronic disorders, including neurodegeneration and cardiomyopathy [1, 2]. It is now apparent that the ocular system is no exception, since numerous eye pathologies are associated with mitochondrial defects as a result of inherited mitochondrial mutations (e.g. Leber's hereditary optic neuropathy, LHON) or cumulative stochastic mitochondrial damage (e.g. age-related macular degeneration, AMD; diabetic retinopathy). Cumulative stochastic injury over a lifetime is not surprising, since the eye is constantly exposed to numerous damaging agents including visible light (in particular the blue region, 475–510 nm), UV (UVA, 320–400 nm) and UVB (280–320 nm) radiation, high concentrations of oxygen, and environmental chemicals (e.g. acrolein from tobacco smoke). This potentially damaging microenvironment strongly favors the generation of reactive oxygen species (ROS), which have the potential to exacerbate mitochondrial mutagenesis and ocular dysfunction [3, 4]. As will be discussed below, cellular ROS can be derived from three main sources: mitochondria, photosensitizers and NADPH oxidase. Elevated mitochondrion-derived ROS have been strongly associated with ocular diseases in both the anterior and posterior

KARGER

Fax +41 61 306 12 34
E-Mail karger@karger.ch
www.karger.com

Accessible online at:
www.karger.com/ore

Michael E. Boulton, PhD
Department of Anatomy and Cell Biology
College of Medicine, University of Florida
PO Box 100235, Gainesville, FL 32610-0235 (USA)
E-Mail meboulton@ufl.edu

segments of the eye [3, 5–7]. In addition, inherited mutations in either mitochondrial genes or nuclear genes encoding mitochondrial proteins result in severe mitochondrial disease causing respiratory chain dysfunction, impairment of replication of mitochondrial DNA (mtDNA) and depletion of mtDNA, which often manifest themselves as disorders of the optic nerve [8–10].

The mitochondrion represents a critical organelle for cellular function and survival. Its principal roles include generation of chemical energy, compartmentalization of cellular metabolism and regulation of programmed cell death. The mitochondria consist of inner and outer membranes composed of phospholipid bilayers containing many integral proteins. The inner membrane is particularly protein rich and is compartmentalized into an inner limiting membrane and complex involutions designated 'cristae' that expand the surface area for ATP production [11]. Encompassed by the inner membrane is the matrix that contains enzymes catalyzing the tricarboxylic acid and urea cycles, fatty acid oxidation, gluconeogenesis as well as committed steps in heme and amino acid synthesis. In addition, the mitochondrial matrix houses the genetic system of the organelle: ribosomes, transfer RNAs (tRNAs) and tRNA synthetases, multiple copies of the mtDNA and the enzymes required for its replication. Given the fact that mitochondria play such an integral role in cellular activity, it is perhaps not surprising that dysfunction can result in a myriad of clinical disorders arising from inherited mutations and/or stochastic ROS-induced genomic injury (fig. 1).

In this review, we outline the mechanistic basis of ROS-induced mtDNA dysfunction and the mitochondrial/oxidative stress theory of aging in relation to the ocular system. In addition, we will discuss the common pathologies associated with mitochondrial dysfunction, with particular emphasis on the role of oxidatively induced and inherited mutations within mtDNA, as causative factors in aging and tissue dysfunctions of the eye.

Mitochondrial and Free Radical Theories of Aging and Disease

The free radical theory of aging was first proposed over 60 years ago, when it was discovered that oxygen radicals were generated in biological systems following exposure to radiation [12, 13]. Harman [14] put forward that oxygen free radicals are formed endogenously during routine metabolism and that they play a pivotal role in the aging process. The discovery of oxidants in vivo and the identification of superoxide dismutase (SOD), an antioxidant whose primary function is to prevent oxidative damage in cells, propelled this principle to the forefront of gerontology theories [15, 16]. In 1972, Harman [17] additionally proposed that mitochondria have a fundamental role in the process of aging. The overall premise of this theory was that ROS generated by the mitochondrial metabolism increase in an age-dependent manner and that ROS-mediated damage to proteins, lipids and mtDNA has a causative role in the morbidity of aging and age-related disease. There are other plausible theories of senescence involving, for example, telomeres and genome stability, but the discovery of the role of sirtuin proteins (a family of proteins that regulate gene silencing and suppress recombination of ribosomal DNA) on mitochondrial function and on extension of life span has refocused attention on the importance of mitochondria in aging [18]. Recent research has demonstrated that mitochondrial deficiencies (either generated by stochastic damage or inherited mutations) are an important cause of cellular degeneration that is associated with ocular dysfunction and aging and have led to the 'mitochondrial-mutation-based' model of ocular degeneration (fig. 2) [19–22]. The cumulative effects of these oxidatively modified mitochondrial components reduce the bioenergetic tone, impair DNA repair, promote ROS production and increase the mtDNA mutation rate.

Inherited Mitochondrial Diseases

The best understood mitochondrial diseases are caused by maternally inherited point mutations or deletions in mtDNA. In addition, mutation of nuclear encoded genes can result in loss of mtDNA stability [23]. Mitochondrial diseases manifest themselves with a broad spectrum of symptoms but frequently affect ocular tissues and often involve heteroplasmy (the coexistence of both mutant and normal mtDNA; fig. 1). Examples include cases of LHON, mitochondrial encephalomyopathy, lactic acidosis and stroke-like episodes (MELAS), chronic progressive external ophthalmoplegia (PEO), and neuropathy, ataxia and retinitis pigmentosa. The symptoms of these disorders range from ophthalmoplegia, optic atrophy, pigmentary retinopathy to macular dystrophy [24].

mtDNA Heteroplasmy

A single mitochondrion may contain 0–21 mtDNA molecules [25, 26]. In healthy cells, the mtDNA molecules are identical, which is termed homoplasmy. Most homo-

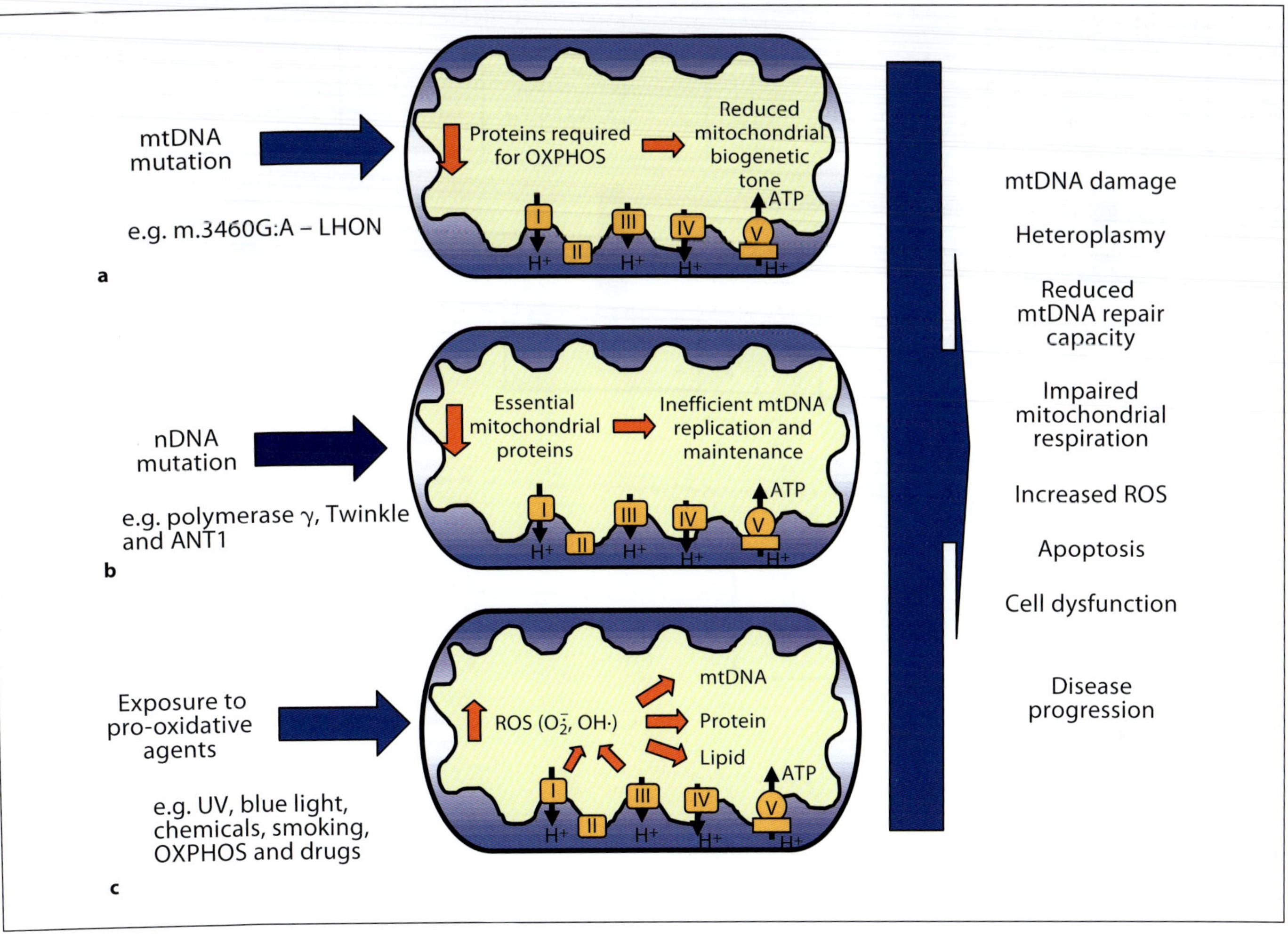

Fig. 1. The role of mtDNA (**a**), nuclear DNA (nDNA) mutations (**b**) and ROS (**c**) in mitochondrial disease. Multiple factors diminish the integrity of mitochondria that lead to loss of cell function, apoptosis and ocular degeneration. **a** The most common mitochondrial diseases, e.g. LHON, result from primary mtDNA mutations that prevent successful completion of respiratory complexes, e.g. complex I, thus reducing mitochondrial oxidative phosphorylation (OXPHOS). **b** Mutations in nDNA-encoded mitochondrial proteins result in an impaired ability to undergo mtDNA replication, maintenance and mtDNA repair. **c** ROS, in particular superoxide (O_2^-), are generated from exposure to exogenous oxidative agents as well as being byproducts of OXPHOS (primarily from complexes I and III of the electron transport chain). ROS damage all mitochondrial macromolecules and include labile Fe-S enzymes such as aconitase which release Fe^{2+} and H_2O_2, promoting Fenton chemistry. The mtDNA is a major target for the hydroxyl radical (OH·) which can lead to increased mutation rates. It is important to note that increased ROS generation is associated with mitochondrial disease irrespective of the causative factor, i.e. mtDNA, nDNA mutation or exogenous oxidative exposure.

plasmic base substitutions are usually found to be neutral polymorphisms, but some homoplasmic mitochondrial DNA mutations such as G11778A in the ND4 gene are an important cause of ocular disease [27, 28]. However, due to the polyploid nature of the mitochondrial genome, wild-type and mutated mtDNA may coexist in an individual mitochondrion, which is referred to as heteroplasmy. Most mtDNA mutations related to diseases are associated with heteroplasmy and can, if within a transcribed mitochondrial gene, affect expression and/or activity of the gene product. In heteroplasmic pedigrees, individuals with a greater amount of mutant mtDNA are at higher risk for visual loss. Typically 80–90% mutant mtDNA is required to produce a clinically observable phenotype. This phenomenon is known as the threshold effect. However, the additional interaction with nuclear-encoded mi-

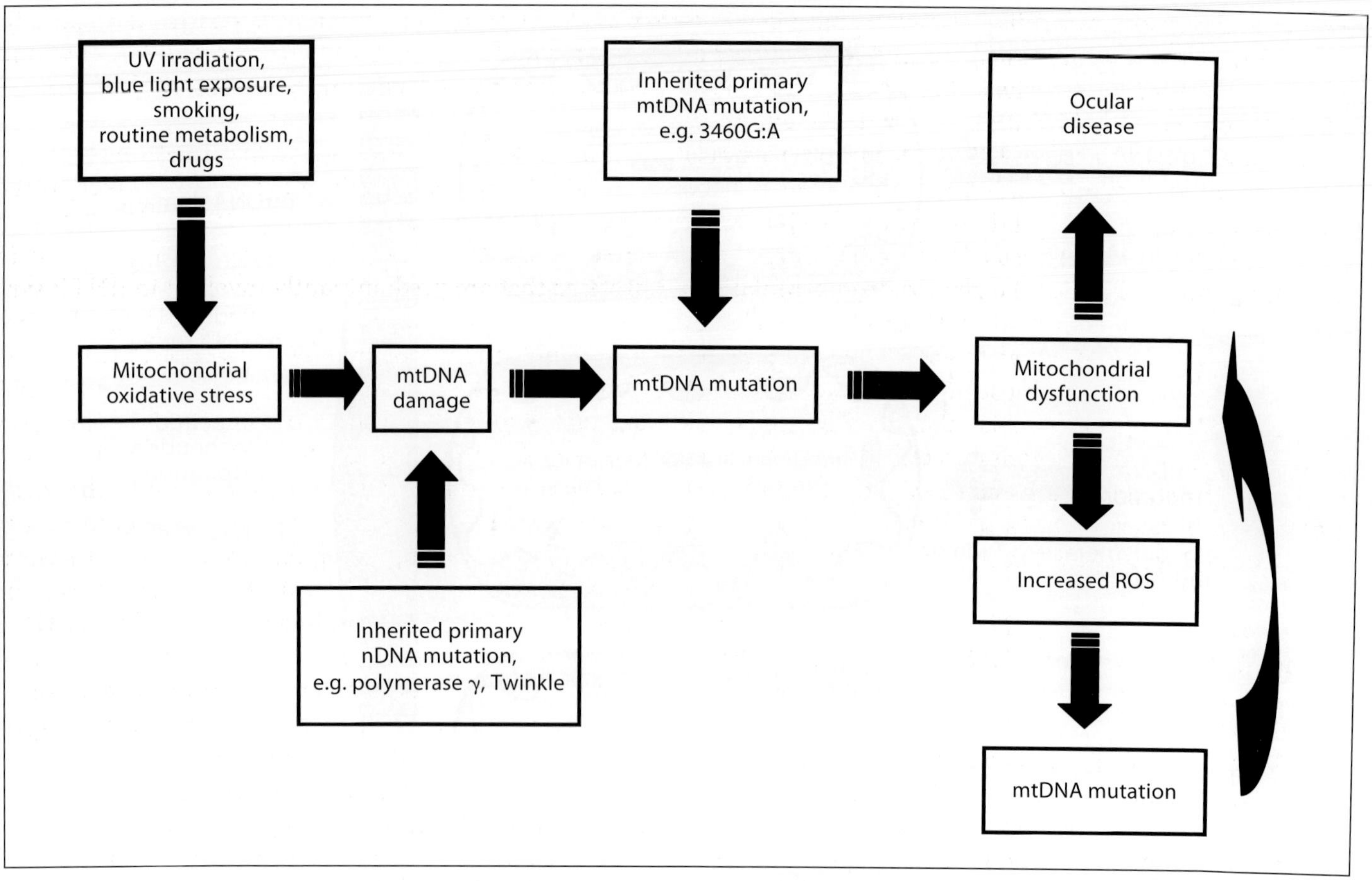

Fig. 2. Mitochondrial-mutation-based model of ocular degeneration. Both mtDNA mutations and nuclear-DNA (nDNA)-encoded mutations in mitochondrial proteins are a primary cause of mitochondrial dysfunction which may in turn be an initiating factor in ocular disease. Intriguingly, mitochondrial oxidative stress (which can be generated from both endogenous and exogenous sources, as well as being a byproduct from mtDNA and nDNA mutations) has a pivotal role in disease progression. After a certain threshold of mitochondrial mutations has been reached, the mitochondria undergo a bioenergetic crisis, resulting in increased ROS and concomitant generation of mtDNA mutations. This causes the level of energy production to drop below that required for cellular functioning, and apoptosis is initiated by the mitochondria, leading to loss of tissue function and contributing to the onset/progression of ocular degeneration.

tochondrial proteins and environmental factors may complicate the issue of assigning a pathogenic role specifically to mtDNA sequence variants. These mutations often undergo mitotic segregation and the levels of normal and mutated mtDNA can vary considerably between cells of the same tissue, a phenomenon that may be influenced by the organization of mtDNA in nucleoids. Mitochondrial heteroplasmy is thought to result in altered proteins that may accumulate over time, thus promoting ocular disease states [6, 29].

mtDNA Mutations

The most common mitochondrial disease with bilateral optic neuropathies is LHON, which results from primary mtDNA mutations affecting the respiratory chain complexes [30, 31]. Over 90% of LHON pedigrees harbor 1 of 3 mtDNA point mutations (m.3460G:A, m.11778G:A, m.14484T:C), all of which affect genes encoding complex I of the respiratory system [32]. Several other mtDNA mutations have been identified with LHON, with most of them also occurring in the respiratory chain [33, 34]. Another mtDNA mutation disorder, MELAS, usually occurs from maternal inheritance, with almost 90% of patients suffering from a mutation at position 3243, encoding the tRNA leucine in mtDNA [35]. Patients with MELAS often have mtDNA deletions and present with retinal pigmentary abnormalities and retinal pigment epithelium (RPE) atrophy similar to those present in the early AMD phenotype [36]. Interestingly, similar symptoms have been associated with some patients with another mitochondrial disorder, maternally inherited diabetes and deafness, which highlights the clinical overlap which often exists with mitochondrial diseases [37, 38]. Neuropathy, ataxia and retinitis pigmentosa syndrome is usually due to the ATP6 T8993G mutation. Children in whom the burden of the mutation exceeds 95% instead succumb to a brainstem disorder known as infantile Leigh's syndrome. Mutations in several of the mitochondrial tRNA genes result in PEO, which is characterized by weakness of the external eye muscles and ptosis. The most common mitochondrial deletion, which causes a multisystem disorder known as Kearns-Sayres syndrome, is associated with the development of retinitis pigmentosa and PEO before the age of 20. Patients with Kearns-Sayres syndrome typically suffer from cardiac conduction defects and cardiomyopathy.

Nuclear DNA Mutations That Affect Mitochondria

Mutations in mitochondrial proteins that are encoded by nuclear DNA (nDNA) also present with ophthalmic manifestations that affect POLG encoding DNA polymerase γ, PEO1 or Twinkle encoding the mtDNA helicase and ANT1 encoding the adenine nucleotide translocator [39–42]. These proteins are required for mtDNA replication, maintenance and repair. Over 80 pathogenic mutations have been documented in DNA polymerase γ (a heterotrimer consisting of a catalytic α- and 2 accessory β-subunits) [43]. It is required for DNA repair as a component in the base excision repair pathway and replication [44]. Mutations in its α-subunit can result in disorders that present as ocular symptoms including sensory-atactic neuropathy, dysarthria and ophthalmoplegia (SANDO) and recessive and sporadic forms of PEO [45]. Twinkle, a hexameric DNA helicase, is generally assumed to be the primary replicative helicase of mtDNA with a 5′ to 3′ polarity and nucleotide triphosphate hydrolase activity. Twinkle interacts with approximately 20 proteins including DNA polymerase γ, to form a component of a replication unit of mtDNA, which helps to explain why mutations in these 2 genes often present in similar manifestations. Over 20 mutations in the Twinkle gene have been associated with PEO, but it has also been described as a recessive mutation in SANDO [46–48]. Mutations in the *ANT1* gene that encodes an adenine nucleotide translocator protein, whose main function is to transport ATP out of the mitochondrial matrix, are also associated with PEO. *ANT1* mutations alter the mitochondrial nucleotide pool which adversely affects mtDNA replication and availability of ADP, thus negatively impacting on the rate of oxidative phosphorylation. Both familial and sporadic missense mutations of ANT1 are thought to occur within the transmembrane domains of the protein [49].

Nucleotide Imbalance and mtDNA Depletion

mtDNA depletion syndrome is a recently recognized disorder involving a quantitative defect of mtDNA. It presents in infancy and is associated with mutations in proteins that are predominantly involved in dNTP synthesis (mitochondrial and cytosolic) including TK2 (encoding mitochondrial thymidine kinase), DGUOK (deoxyguanosine kinase) and SUCLA1 and 2 (α- and β-subunit of the mitochondrial matrix enzyme succinyl-CoA synthetase) among others [50–52]. Constant supplies of dNTPs are crucial for the maintenance of mitochondrial genomic integrity, which are either supplied by import of cytosolic dNTPs or by salvaging deoxynucleosides within mitochondria. Alterations in the cellular nucleotide pool generate a promutagenic state and inefficient DNA repair and synthesis propagating mitochondrial mutagenesis [53]. The first identified mitochondrial disease associated with the dNTP pool is mitochondrial neurogastrointestinal encephalomyopathy (MNGIE), which is characterized by ocular defects such as ophthalmoplegia and pigmentary retinopathy [54]. It is of further interest to note that nucleotide imbalance, such as that observed in MNGIE, is highly mutagenic and has the potential to impair the DNA repair processes [55].

Mitochondrially Generated ROS

Mitochondria account for the bulk of endogenously formed ROS in most cells [17, 56, 57] with the mitochondrial respiratory chain acting as the major intracellular source of ROS [58–60]. An unavoidable respiratory electron leak from complexes I and III results in the formation of superoxide, O_2^-, which can react with lipids, protein and DNA [61–64]. The O_2^- can be readily converted into H_2O_2 either spontaneously or via a dismutation reaction involving manganese superoxide dismutase (MnSOD), a resident of the mitochondrial matrix. In the presence of redox active metal ions, H_2O_2 may, via the Fenton reaction, generate the highly reactive hydroxyl radical (OH•) [56]. The OH• radical is responsible for multiple sites of mtDNA damage including single- and double-strand breaks, abasic sites and base modifications.

A further oxidative burden is caused by damage induced by O_2^- to Fe-S centers of mitochondrial proteins and includes subunits of complexes I, II and III as well as aconitase [65–67]. Labile Fe-S enzymes such as mitochondrial aconitase, offer an important target for ROS. Of particular relevance to the eye, mitochondria located in cells exposed to visible light generate ROS via interactions with mitochondrial photosensitizers, like cytochrome c oxidase, to generate ROS and mtDNA damage [68, 69]. The transfer of energy from photoactivated chromophores to oxygen leads to the formation of singlet oxygen, $^1O_2$, which exists in an excited state. $^1O_2$ can generate ROS such as O_2^- by interacting with diatomic oxygen and by reacting directly with electrons with double bonds without the formation of free radical intermediates [70].

It is also important to note that specific tissues within the eye can also generate significant levels of ROS from nonmitochondrial sources. For example, lipofuscin (an age-related pigment that accumulates in RPE cells with age) is a potent photoinducible generator of ROS, and, in microvascular endothelial cells, NADPH oxidase is considered to be a major source of superoxide. Studies suggest that these ROS can also contribute to exogenous oxidative damage of the mitochondria, thus exacerbating mitochondrial dysfunction [69, 71, 72].

Mitochondrial Genome

Mitochondria are semiautonomous organelles that contain multiple copies of the 16,569-bp circular mtDNA. The mitochondrial genome encodes 37 genes, with 13 genes encoding protein subunits of the electron transport chain, and 24 genes encoding tRNAs and ribosomal RNAs needed for protein synthesis [73]. Moreover, a noncoding region referred to as the displacement loop or regulatory region is required for initiation of transcription and DNA synthesis. This noncoding region contains 2 hypervariable segments (HVS-I and HVS-II) with high polymorphism [74, 75]. The replication and repair of the mitochondrial genome are distinct from those of the nucleus and continue in postmitotic cells, such as the RPE and photoreceptors. The maintenance and repair of mtDNA are completely dependent upon proteins transcribed by the nuclear genome. mtDNA is organized into nucleoprotein complexes known as nucleoids that contain proteins directly bound to the DNA and which appear to associate mtDNA with the inner mitochondrial membrane [76]. It is generally assumed that the mtDNA is more sensitive to ROS and other chemicals compared to the nDNA [77].

mtDNA Damage and Repair

The stability of the mitochondrial genome is frequently challenged by endogenous and exogenous agents, including ROS which constitute the major endogenous source of mtDNA damage. mtDNA is particularly vulnerable to oxidative damage, due in part to its close proximity to the inner mitochondrial membrane where the majority of the ROS are generated and the fact that it does not contain histones which are thought to act as a physical barrier against ROS in the nuclear genome [6]. Furthermore it appears that oxidative damage to mtDNA is more extensive and persists longer compared to nDNA damage [77]. Such ROS-induced mtDNA damage includes base modifications, abasic sites, strand breaks and bulky adducts as well as a number of covalent modifications to DNA, which encompass single-nucleobase lesions, strand breaks, inter- and intrastrand cross-links, along with protein-DNA cross-links [78, 79]. The most studied oxidative lesion, 8-oxo-2′-deoxyguanosine, is capable of pairing with an adenine as well as cytosine during DNA replication, thus resulting in a G:C-to-T:A transversion mutation after 2 rounds of replication. Interestingly, levels of 8-oxo-2′-deoxyguanosine are greater in the mtDNA compared to the nDNA and are strongly correlated with large-scale mitochondrial deletions [80].

Mitochondria have less capacity for DNA repair than do nuclei [77, 81], and this is exacerbated by components of the mtDNA repair pathway being sensitive to oxidative inactivation [82]. Although the nucleotide excision repair pathway and recombination repair are absent in mitochondria, it is now known that mitochondria do indeed possess multiple alternative DNA repair pathways [6]. Oxidative mtDNA damage is thought to be repaired primarily by base excision repair [6, 83–86]. Double-strand break repair and mismatch repair have also been recently reported to be active in the mitochondria [87, 88]. DNA repair enzymes that are active against alkylated bases have also been identified within the mitochondrial compartment, and alkylated mtDNA is efficiently repaired in the mitochondria [6, 84, 89]. Thus, as the mtDNA molecule is highly susceptible to ROS-induced damage and mtDNA integrity is critical for cell survival, it is not surprising that multiple DNA repair pathways have evolved within the mitochondria [90]. The fact that each mitochondrion contains multiple copies of mtDNA also provides a significant measure of protection, given that heteroplasmic mutations do not lead to mitochondrial malfunction until they become the predominant species (see below).

Stochastic Mitochondrial Damage and Ocular Degeneration

Ocular tissues, including the retina, the optic nerve, photoreceptor cells and lens, exist in highly oxidizing microenvironments that are subjected to constant damaging light and/or UV wavelengths together with high oxygen fluxes, which strongly promote oxidative damage [4, 69, 91, 92]. Furthermore, environmental insults such as smoking add to the level of oxidative stress [93]. Research over the last few decades has provided compelling evidence of oxidative-stress-induced damage to mitochondria affecting protein, lipid and DNA and that resultant mitochondrial dysfunction contributes to the pathogenesis of several ocular disease(s) and in the aging process itself [4, 6, 92, 94] (fig. 1, 2). Because animal mitochondria are deficient in nucleotide and excision repair pathways [77], stochastic mtDNA defects can remain for life leading to the concept of 'metabolic memory' [95].

Age-Related Macular Degeneration

There is now strong support for mitochondrial genomic dysfunction being involved in AMD from clinical studies and animal models. There is a significant decrease in number and area of RPE mitochondria with increasing age, and these age-related changes are significantly increased in the eyes of AMD donors [96]. Recently, mtDNA haplogroups have been identified that are associated with either increased or decreased prevalence of age-related maculopathy [97–99]. These findings suggest that the bioenergetic consequences of mtDNA derangements may be expressed in macular RPE as a maculopathy or contribute to the development of AMD. A strong association between a variant of LOC387715/ARMS2 and AMD has been reported [100, 101]. Early reports suggested that ARMS2 is a mitochondrial protein, though these results have been questioned [102].

Evidence from a number of studies now strongly supports that mitochondrial dysfunction initiated by mtDNA damage is a feature that underlies the development of retinal aging and AMD. Increased mtDNA deletions have been documented in aged human and rodent retinas [103, 104] and increased mtDNA damage and decreased repair are associated with aging and AMD [104, 105]. Furthermore, the repair of the RPE mitochondrial genome appears to be slow and relatively inefficient [106]. Photoreceptor outer segments have been shown to damage RPE mtDNA in vitro, by a burst of ROS generated during ingestion. Blue light exposure also harms mitochondrial respiratory activity and damages mtDNA [69]. In addition, a recent report shows that the aged RPE and choroid of rodents suffer extensive mtDNA damage and that this is likely to be due to decreased DNA repair capability [104]. Changes in selected redox proteins and proteins involved in mitochondrial trafficking [107–109] and a decrease in RPE mitochondrial respiration also correlate with AMD progression [105]. Knockdown of MnSOD, the mitochondrial antioxidant responsible for neutralizing superoxide anions, results in pathological lesions in mice similar to those observed in 'dry' AMD [110]. Ex vivo studies show that RPE cells exposed to high levels of ROS suffer preferential damage to mtDNA and subsequent repair is poor [89, 111, 112].

Uveitis

Intraocular inflammation, commonly referred to as uveitis, is a principal causative factor underlying blindness from retinal photoreceptor degeneration. Oxidative retinal damage in uveitis is caused by activated macrophages, which generate various cytotoxic agents, including inducible nitric oxide produced by inducible nitric oxide synthase, O_2^- and other ROS [113]. Oxidative stress plays an important role in the photoreceptor mitochondria during the early phase of experimental autoimmune uveitis (EAU). It has been shown that mtDNA damage occurs early in EAU; interestingly, nDNA damage occurred later in EAU [5]. Furthermore, mitochondrial proteins in the photoreceptor inner segments are modified by peroxynitrite-mediated nitration [114] which, in turn, leads to increased generation of mitochondrial ROS. In support of an increased state of mitochondrial oxidative stress, MnSOD has been shown to be upregulated during EAU, presumably to counteract ROS [115]. Recent data appear to suggest a causative role of oxidative mtDNA damage in the early phase of EAU, before leukocyte infiltration. Such oxidative damage in the mitochondria may be the initial event leading to retinal degeneration in uveitis [5].

Glaucoma

Increasingly persuasive evidence suggests that glaucomatous tissue damage initiated by elevated intraocular pressure and/or tissue hypoxia also involves oxidative stress. Experimental elevation of intraocular pressure induces oxidative stress in the retina. It also appears that mitochondrial oxidative stress may have an important role in glaucomatous neurodegeneration [116–118]. In glaucoma there is evidence that mitochondrial dysfunction may lower the bioenergetic state of retinal ganglion cells leading to an increased susceptibility to oxidative stress and apoptotic cell death [118, 119]. In addition, light exposure may be an oxidative risk factor, whereby it reduces mitochondrial function and increases ROS production in ganglion cells [120]. Mitochondrial dysfunction has also been implicated in neuronal apoptosis in experimental models of glaucoma [121, 122]. mtDNA abnormalities further support a role of mitochondrial-dysfunction-associated stress as a risk factor for glaucoma patients [123].

Diabetic Retinopathy

Mitochondrial dysfunction has been shown to play an important role in diabetic retinopathy [94, 118]. Retinal mitochondria experience increased oxidative stress in diabetes, and complex III is one of the major sources of the increased O_2^- [124]. Superoxide levels are elevated in the retina of diabetic rats and in retinal vascular endothelial cells incubated in high-glucose media [125], and hydrogen peroxide content is increased in the retina of diabetic rats [126]. Membrane lipid peroxidation and oxidative damage to DNA, the consequences of ROS-induced injury, are elevated in the retina in diabetes [127]. Chronic overproduction of ROS in the retina results in aberrant mitochondrial functions in diabetes [94], and hyperglycemia-induced overproduction of superoxide by the mitochondrial electron transport chain is considered to activate the major pathways of hyperglycemic damage by inhibiting GAPDH activity. However, the mechanism by which hyperglycemia causes an increase in mitochondrial ROS is not yet fully understood, with some implicating a direct effect and others an indirect role via high-glucose-induced cytokines [128–131]. Elevated O_2^- levels activate caspase 3 which leads to cell death in the retinal capillaries [94]. Upregulation of SOD2 inhibited diabetes-induced increases in mitochondrial O_2^-, restored mitochondrial function and prevented vascular pathology both in vitro and in vivo [124, 132–134]. However, timing of such treatments is critical since animal studies have demonstrated that oxidative stress contributes not only to the development of diabetic retinopathy, but also to the resistance of retinopathy to reversal after good glycemic control has been reinstituted – the metabolic memory phenomenon [135]. Resistance of diabetic retinopathy to reversal is possibly attributable to accumulation of damaged molecules in mitochondria and ROS-induced damage that is not easily removed even after good glycemic control has been reestablished. However, the accumulation of advanced glycation end products is also implicated in metabolic memory [136].

Variation in mtDNA has also been linked to resistance to type 1 diabetes. A single nucleotide change (C5173A), resulting in a leucine-to-methionine amino acid substitution in the mitochondrially encoded NADH dehydrogenase subunit 2 gene, is associated with resistance to type 1 diabetes in a Japanese population [137]. Similarly, an orthologous polymorphism (C4738A), resulting in an L-to-M substitution, provides resistance against the development of spontaneous diabetes compared with the diabetes-prone nonobese diabetic mouse strain [138]. Gusdon et al. [139] have shown that the methionine substitution results in a lower level of ROS production from complex III.

Cataract

Oxidative stress plays a significant role in cataractogenesis [92, 140]. The lens is highly susceptible to ROS, and mitochondria are located in the epithelium and superficial fiber cells. Interestingly, in these cell types, the mitochondria have been confirmed as the major source of ROS generation [141]. Several in vitro studies have demonstrated that human lens cells are highly susceptible to oxidative insults, in which antioxidant activity is generally inversely proportional to cataract severity [142]. Oxidation of proteins, lipids and DNA has been observed in cataractous lenses [143–145]. Proteins from cataractous lenses lose sulfhydryl groups, contain oxidized residues, generate high-molecular-weight aggregates and become insoluble [140]. In addition, cataract has been shown to be a symptom of a newly identified mitochondrial disease called autosomal-recessive myopathy, caused by mutations in the growth factor, augmenter of liver regeneration gene, which affects protein levels of the mitochondrial intermembrane space [146].

Conclusion

The findings discussed highlight the importance of mtDNA damage arising from both stochastic ROS and maternally inherited mutations. mtDNA genomic instability is a principal defect in the etiology of multiple diseases that result in ocular manifestations (summarized in fig. 2). Continued research in this clinically relevant area will undoubtedly provide a greater understanding of how deficiencies/failure of the mitochondrial genome contribute to the pathogenesis of degenerative diseases. Future challenges will involve developing therapeutic strategies that target mitochondria and manipulate mtDNA replication, repair and levels of nucleotide precursors to maintain mtDNA integrity with the ultimate goal of blocking or retarding the effects of mitochondrial disease.

Acknowledgement

This work was supported by NIH grant EY019688.

References

1 Monsalve M, Borniquel S, Valle I, Lamas S:Mitochondrial dysfunction in human pathologies. Front Biosci 2007;12:1131–1153.
2 Reeve AK, Krishnan KJ, Turnbull D: Mitochondrial DNA mutations in disease, aging, and neurodegeneration. Ann NY Acad Sci 2008;1147:21–29.
3 Beatty S, Koh H, Phil M, Henson D, Boulton M:The role of oxidative stress in the pathogenesis of age-related macular degeneration. Surv Ophthalmol 2000;45:115–134.
4 Ohia SE, Opere CA, Leday AM: Pharmacological consequences of oxidative stress in ocular tissues. Mutat Res 2005;579:22–36.
5 Khurana RN, Parikh JG, Saraswathy S, Wu GS, Rao NA:Mitochondrial oxidative DNA damage in experimental autoimmune uveitis. Invest Ophthalmol Vis Sci 2008;49:3299–3304.
6 Jarrett SG, Lin H, Godley BF, Boulton ME:Mitochondrial DNA damage and its potential role in retinal degeneration. Prog Retin Eye Res 2008;27:596–607.
7 Green K:Free radicals and aging of anterior segment tissues of the eye: a hypothesis. Ophthalmic Res 1995;27(suppl 1):143–149.
8 Carelli V, La Morgia C, Iommarini L, Carroccia R, Mattiazzi M, Sangiorgi S, Farne S, Maresca A, Foscarini B, Lanzi L, Amadori M, Bellan M, Valentino ML: Mitochondrial optic neuropathies:how two genomes may kill the same cell type? Biosci Rep 2007;27: 173–184.
9 Carelli V, Ross-Cisneros FN, Sadun AA: Mitochondrial dysfunction as a cause of optic neuropathies. Prog Retinal Eye Res 2004; 23:53–89.
10 Copeland WC:Inherited mitochondrial diseases of DNA replication. Annu Rev Med 2008;59:131–146.
11 Mannella CA:The relevance of mitochondrial membrane topology to mitochondrial function. Biochim Biophys Acta 2006;1762: 140–147.
12 Gerschman R, Gilbert DL, Nye SW, Dwyer P, Fenn WO:Oxygen poisoning and X-irradiation:a mechanism in common. Science 1954;119:623–626.
13 Gerschman R, Gilbert DL, Nye SW, Fenn WO: Influence of X-irradiation on oxygen poisoning in mice. Proc Soc Exp Biol Med 1954;86:27–29.
14 Harman D:Aging: a theory based on free radical and radiation chemistry. J Gerontol 1956;11:298–300.
15 McCord JM, Fridovich I: Superoxide dismutase:an enzymic function for erythrocuprein (hemocuprein). J Biol Chem 1969; 244:6049–6055.
16 McCord JM, Fridovich I: The utility of superoxide dismutase in studying free radical reactions. I. Radicals generated by the interaction of sulfite, dimethyl sulfoxide, and oxygen. J Biol Chem 1969;244:6056–6063.
17 Harman D: The biologic clock: the mitochondria? J Am Geriatr Soc 1972;20:145–147.
18 Guarente L: Mitochondria – a nexus for aging, calorie restriction, and sirtuins? Cell 2008;132:171–176.
19 Coleman HR, Chan CC, Ferris FL 3rd, Chew EY: Age-related macular degeneration. Lancet 2008;372:1835–1845.
20 Williams DL: Oxidative stress and the eye. Vet Clin North Am 2008;38:179–192.
21 Santosa S, Jones PJ: Oxidative stress in ocular disease: does lutein play a protective role? Can Med Assoc J 2005;173:861–862.
22 O'Connor GR: Factors related to the initiation and recurrence of uveitis: Xlth Edward Jackson Memorial Lecture. Am J Ophthalmol 1983;96:577–599.
23 Thorburn DR: Mitochondrial disorders: prevalence, myths and advances. J Inherit Metab Dis 2004;27:349–362.
24 Johns DR: The ophthalmologic manifestations of mitochondrial disease. Semin Ophthalmol 1995;10:295–302.
25 Cavelier L, Johannisson A, Gyllensten U: Analysis of mtDNA copy number and composition of single mitochondrial particles using flow cytometry and PCR. Exp Cell Res 2000;259:79–85.
26 Satoh M, Kuroiwa T: Organization of multiple nucleoids and DNA molecules in mitochondria of a human cell. Exp Cell Res 1991; 196:137–140.
27 Kerrison JB, Howell N, Miller NR, Hirst L, Green WR: Leber hereditary optic neuropathy: electron microscopy and molecular genetic analysis of a case. Ophthalmology 1995;102:1509–1516.
28 Di Mauro S, Schon EA: Mitochondrial disorders in the nervous system. Annu Rev Neurosci 2008;31:91–123.
29 Puomila A, Viitanen T, Savontaus ML, Nikoskelainen E, Huoponen K: Segregation of the nd4/11778 and the nd1/3460 mutations in four heteroplasmic LHON families. J Neurol Sci 2002;205:41–45.
30 Carelli V, Sadun AA: Optic neuropathy in LHON and Leigh syndrome. Ophthalmology 2001;108:1172–1173.
31 Carelli V, Valentino ML, Liguori R, Meletti S, Vetrugno R, Provini F, Mancardi GL, Bandini F, Baruzzi A, Montagna P: Leber's hereditary optic neuropathy (LHON/11778) with myoclonus: report of two cases. J Neurol Neurosurg Psychiatry 2001;71:813–816.
32 Mackey DA, Oostra RJ, Rosenberg T, Nikoskelainen E, Bronte-Stewart J, Poulton J, Harding AE, Govan G, Bolhuis PA, Norby S: Primary pathogenic mtDNA mutations in multigeneration pedigrees with Leber hereditary optic neuropathy. Am J Hum Genet 1996;59:481–485.
33 Howell N, Halvorson S, Burns J, McCullough DA, Paulton J: When does bilateral optic atrophy become Leber hereditary optic neuropathy? Am J Hum Genet 1993;53:959–963.
34 Besch D, Wissinger B, Zrenner E, Leo-Kotter B: A case of Leber optic neuropathy with a new point mutation in the cytochrome b gene. Ophthalmologe 2000;97:22–26.
35 Sproule DM, Kaufmann P: Mitochondrial encephalopathy, lactic acidosis, and stroke-like episodes: basic concepts, clinical phenotype, and therapeutic management of MELAS syndrome. Ann NY Acad Sci 2008; 1142:133–158.
36 Jones M, Mitchell P, Wang JJ, Sue C: MELAS A3243G mitochondrial DNA mutation and age related maculopathy. Am J Ophthalmol 2004;138:1051–1053.
37 Kokotas H, Petersen MB, Willems PJ: Mitochondrial deafness. Clin Genet 2007;71:379–391.
38 Laloi-Michelin M, Meas T, Ambonville C, Bellanne-Chantelot C, Beaufils S, Massin P, Vialettes B, Gin H, Timsit J, Bauduceau B, Bernard L, Bertin E, Blickle JF, Cahen-Varsaux J, Cailleba A, Casanova S, Cathebras P, Charpentier G, Chedin P, Crea T, Delemer B, Dubois-Laforgue D, Duchemin F, Ducluzeau PH, Bouhanick B, Dusselier L, Gabreau T, Grimaldi A, Guerci B, Jacquin V, Kaloustian E, Larger E, Lecleire-Collet A, Lorenzini F, Louis J, Mausset J, Murat A, Nadler-Fluteau S, Olivier F, Paquis-Flucklinger V, Paris-Bockel D, Raynaud I, Reznik Y, Riveline JP, Schneebeli S, Sonnet E, Sola-Gazagnes A, Thomas JL, Trabulsi B, Virally M, Guillausseau PJ: The clinical variability of maternally inherited diabetes and deafness is associated with the degree of heteroplasmy in blood leukocytes. J Clin Endocrinol Metab 2009;94:3025–3030.

39 Chan SS, Longley MJ, Copeland WC: Modulation of the W748S mutation in DNA polymerase gamma by the E1143G polymorphism in mitochondrial disorders. Hum Mol Genet 2006;15:3473–3483.
40 Graziewicz MA, Bienstock RJ, Copeland WC: The DNA polymerase gamma Y955C disease variant associated with PEO and parkinsonism mediates the incorporation and translesion synthesis opposite 7,8-dihydro-8-oxo-2'-deoxyguanosine. Hum Mol Genet 2007;16:2729–2739.
41 Goffart S, Cooper HM, Tyynismaa H, Wanrooij S, Suomalainen A, Spelbrink JN: Twinkle mutations associated with autosomal dominant progressive external ophthalmoplegia lead to impaired helicase function and in vivo mtDNA replication stalling. Hum Mol Genet 2009;18:328–340.
42 Lim SE, Ponamarev MV, Longley MJ, Copeland WC: Structural determinants in human DNA polymerase gamma account for mitochondrial toxicity from nucleoside analogs. J Mol Biol 2003;329:45–57.
43 Graziewicz MA, Longley MJ, Copeland WC: DNA polymerase gamma in mitochondrial DNA replication and repair. Chem Rev 2006;106:383–405.
44 Bohr VA: Repair of oxidative DNA damage in nuclear and mitochondrial DNA, and some changes with aging in mammalian cells. Free Radic Biol Med 2002;32:804–812.
45 Hudson G, Chinnery PF: Mitochondrial DNA polymerase-gamma and human disease. Hum Mol Genet 2006;15(spec No 2): R244–R252.
46 Van Hove JL, Cunningham V, Rice C, Ringel SP, Zhang Q, Chou PC, Truong CK, Wong LJ: Finding twinkle in the eyes of a 71-year-old lady: a case report and review of the genotypic and phenotypic spectrum of twinkle-related dominant disease. Am J Med Genet 2009;149A:861–867.
47 Liu Z, Ding Y, Du A, Zhang B, Zhao G, Ding M: A novel twinkle (PEO1) gene mutation in a Chinese family with ADPEO. Mol Vis 2008;14:1995–2001.
48 Gago MF, Rosas MJ, Guimaraes J, Ferreira M, Vilarinho L, Castro L, Carpenter S: SANDO: two novel mutations in POLG1 gene. Neuromuscul Disord 2006;16:507–509.
49 Agostino A, Valletta L, Chinnery PF, Ferrari G, Carrara F, Taylor RW, Schaefer AM, Turnbull DM, Tiranti V, Zeviani M: Mutations of ANT1, twinkle, and POLG1 in sporadic progressive external ophthalmoplegia (PEO). Neurology 2003;60:1354–1356.
50 Saada A, Shaag A, Mandel H, Nevo Y, Eriksson S, Elpeleg O: Mutant mitochondrial thymidine kinase in mitochondrial DNA depletion myopathy. Nat Genet 2001;29:342–344.
51 Elpeleg O, Miller C, Hershkovitz E, Bitner-Glindzicz M, Bondi-Rubinstein G, Rahman S, Pagnamenta A, Eshhar S, Saada A: Deficiency of the ADP-forming succinyl-CoA synthase activity is associated with encephalomyopathy and mitochondrial DNA depletion. Am J Hum Genet 2005;76:1081–1086.
52 Mandel H, Szargel R, Labay V, Elpeleg O, Saada A, Shalata A, Anbinder Y, Berkowitz D, Hartman C, Barak M, Eriksson S, Cohen N: The deoxyguanosine kinase gene is mutated in individuals with depleted hepatocerebral mitochondrial DNA. Nat Genet 2001; 29:337–341.
53 Ashley N, Adams S, Slama A, Zeviani M, Suomalainen A, Andreu AL, Naviaux RK, Poulton J: Defects in maintenance of mitochondrial DNA are associated with intramitochondrial nucleotide imbalances. Hum Mol Genet 2007;16:1400–1411.
54 Bedlack RS, Vu T, Hammans S, Sparr SA, Myers B, Morgenlander J, Hirano M: MNGIE neuropathy: five cases mimicking chronic inflammatory demyelinating polyneuropathy. Muscle Nerve 2004;29:364–368.
55 Burkhalter MD, Roberts SA, Havener JM, Ramsden DA: Activity of ribonucleotide reductase helps determine how cells repair DNA double strand breaks. DNA Repair 2009;8:1258–1263.
56 Halliwell B, Gutteridge JM: Free Radicals in Biology and Medicine. New York, Oxford University Press, 1999.
57 Terman A, Brunk UT: Oxidative stress, accumulation of biological 'garbage', and aging. Antioxid Redox Signal 2006;8:197–204.
58 Beckman KB, Ames BN: The free radical theory of aging matures. Physiol Rev 1998; 78:547–581.
59 Beckman KB, Ames BN: Mitochondrial aging:open questions. Ann NY Acad Sci 1998;854:118–127.
60 Lee HC, Wei YH:Oxidative stress, mitochondrial DNA mutation, and apoptosis in aging. Exp Biol Med (Maywood) 2007;232: 592–606.
61 Brand MD, Affourtit C, Esteves TC, Green K, Lambert AJ, Miwa S, Pakay JL, Parker N: Mitochondrial superoxide: production, biological effects, and activation of uncoupling proteins. Free Radic Biol Med 2004;37:755–767.
62 Estabrook RW: Observations on the antimycin A inhibition of biological oxidations. II. Electronic analog computer studies. Biochim Biophys Acta 1962;60:249–258.
63 Cadenas E, Davies KJ: Mitochondrial free radical generation, oxidative stress, and aging. Free Radic Biol Med 2000;29:222–230.
64 Turrens JF, Alexandre A, Lehninger AL: Ubisemiquinone is the electron donor for superoxide formation by complex III of heart mitochondria. Arch Biochem Biophys 1985; 237:408–414.
65 Fridovich I: Superoxide anion radical (O_2^-), superoxide dismutases, and related matters. J Biol Chem 1997;272:18515–18517.
66 Patel M, Day BJ, Crapo JD, Fridovich I, McNamara JO: Requirement for superoxide in excitotoxic cell death. Neuron 1996;16:345–355.
67 Liang LP, Patel M: Iron-sulfur enzyme mediated mitochondrial superoxide toxicity in experimental Parkinson's disease. J Neurochem 2004;90:1076–1084.
68 Chen E, Soderberg PG, Lindstrom B: Cytochrome oxidase activity in rat retina after exposure to 404 nm blue light. Curr Eye Res 1992;11:825–831.
69 Godley BF, Shamsi FA, Liang FQ, Jarrett SG, Davies S, Boulton M: Blue light induces mitochondrial DNA damage and free radical production in epithelial cells. J Biol Chem 2005;280:21061–21066.
70 Min DB, Boff JM: Chemistry and reaction of singlet oxygen in foods. Comp Rev Food Sci Food Safety 2002;1:58–72.
71 Newsholme P, Haber EP, Hirabara SM, Rebelato EL, Procopio J, Morgan D, Oliveira-Emilio HC, Carpinelli AR, Curi R: Diabetes associated cell stress and dysfunction: role of mitochondrial and non-mitochondrial ROS production and activity. J Physiol 2007;583:9–24.
72 Whiteside CI: Cellular mechanisms and treatment of diabetes vascular complications converge on reactive oxygen species. Curr Hypertens Rep 2005;7:148–154.
73 Attardi G, Schatz G: Biogenesis of mitochondria. Annu Rev Cell Biol 1988;4:289–333.
74 Howell N, Bindoff LA, McCullough DA, Kubacka I, Poulton J, Mackey D, Taylor L, Turnbull DM: Leber hereditary optic neuropathy: identification of the same mitochondrial ND1 mutation in six pedigrees. Am J Hum Genet 1991;49:939–950.
75 Shafa Shariat Panahi M, Houshmand M, Tabassi AR: Mitochondrial D-loop variation in Leber hereditary neuropathy patients harboring primary G11778A, G3460A, T14484C mutations: J and W haplogroups as high-risk factors. Arch Med Res 2006;37:1028–1033.
76 Holt IJ, He J, Mao CC, Boyd-Kirkup JD, Martinsson P, Sembongi H, Reyes A, Spelbrink JN: Mammalian mitochondrial nucleoids: organizing an independently minded genome. Mitochondrion 2007;7:311–321.
77 Yakes FM, Van Houten B: Mitochondrial DNA damage is more extensive and persists longer than nuclear DNA damage in human cells following oxidative stress. Proc Natl Acad Sci USA 1997;94:514–519.
78 Bohr VA, Ottersen OP, Tonjum T: Genome instability and DNA repair in brain, ageing and neurological disease. Neuroscience 2007;145:1183–1186.
79 Breen AP, Murphy JA: Reactions of oxyl radicals with DNA. Free Radic Biol Med 1995; 18:1033–1077.

80 Richter C, Park JW, Ames BN: Normal oxidative damage to mitochondrial and nuclear DNA is extensive. Proc Natl Acad Sci USA 1988;85:6465–6467.
81 Ballinger SW, Patterson C, Yan CN, Doan R, Burow DL, Young CG, Yakes FM, Van Houten B, Ballinger CA, Freeman BA, Runge MS: Hydrogen peroxide- and peroxynitrite-induced mitochondrial DNA damage and dysfunction in vascular endothelial and smooth muscle cells. Circ Res 2000;86:960–966.
82 Graziewicz MA, Day BJ, Copeland WC: The mitochondrial DNA polymerase as a target of oxidative damage. Nucleic Acids Res 2002;30:2817–2824.
83 Harrison JF, Hollensworth SB, Spitz DR, Copeland WC, Wilson GL, Le Doux SP: Oxidative stress-induced apoptosis in neurons correlates with mitochondrial DNA base excision repair pathway imbalance. Nucleic Acids Res 2005;33:4660–4671.
84 Le Doux SP, Wilson GL, Beecham EJ, Stevnsner T, Wassermann K, Bohr VA: Repair of mitochondrial DNA after various types of DNA damage in Chinese hamster ovary cells. Carcinogenesis 1992;13:1967–1973.
85 Stuart JA, Mayard S, Hashiguchi K, Souza-Pinto NC, Bohr VA: Localization of mitochondrial DNA base excision repair to an inner membrane-associated particulate fraction. Nucleic Acids Res 2005;33:3722–3732.
86 Tomkinson AE, Bonk RT, Kim J, Bartfeld N, Linn S: Mammalian mitochondrial endonuclease activities specific for ultraviolet-irradiated DNA. Nucleic Acids Res 1990;18:929–935.
87 Mason PA, Matheson EC, Hall AG, Lightowlers RN: Mismatch repair activity in mammalian mitochondria. Nucleic Acids Res 2003;31:1052–1058.
88 Abner CW, McKinnon PJ: The DNA double-strand break response in the nervous system. DNA Repair (Amst) 2004;3:1141–1147.
89 Jarrett SG, Boulton ME: Poly(ADP-ribose) polymerase offers protection against oxidative and alkylation damage to the nuclear and mitochondrial genomes of the retinal pigment epithelium. Ophthalmic Res 2007; 39:213–223.
90 Grishko VI, Rachek LI, Spitz DR, Wilson GL, Le Doux SP: Contribution of mitochondrial DNA repair to cell resistance from oxidative stress. J Biol Chem 2005;280:8901–8905.
91 Liang FQ, Alssadi R, Morehead P, Awasthi YC, Godley BF: Enhanced expression of glutathione-S-transferase A1-1 protects against oxidative stress in human retinal pigment epithelial cells. Exp Eye Res 2005;80:113–119.
92 Brennan LA, Kantorow M: Mitochondrial function and redox control in the aging eye:role of MSRA and other repair systems in cataract and macular degenerations. Exp Eye Res 2009;88:195–203.
93 Tomany SC, Wang JJ, Van Leeuwen R, Klein R, Mitchell P, Vingerling JR, Klein BE, Smith W, De Jong PT: Risk factors for incident age-related macular degeneration: pooled findings from 3 continents. Ophthalmology 2004;111:1280–1287.
94 Kowluru RA:Diabetic retinopathy: mitochondrial dysfunction and retinal capillary cell death. Antioxid Redox Signal 2005;7: 1581–1587.
95 Kowluru RA, Chan PS:Metabolic memory in diabetes – from in vitro oddity to in vivo problem: role of apoptosis. Brain Res Bull 20010;81:297–302.
96 Feher J, Kovacs I, Artico M, Cavallotti C, Papale A, Balacco Gabrieli C: Mitochondrial alterations of retinal pigment epithelium in age-related macular degeneration. Neurobiol Aging 2006;27:983–993.
97 Jones MM, Manwaring N, Wang JJ, Rochtchina E, Mitchell P, Sue CM: Mitochondrial DNA haplogroups and age-related maculopathy. Arch Ophthalmol 2007; 125:1235–1240.
98 Udar N, Atilano SR, Memarzadeh M, Boyer DS, Chwa M, Lu S, Maguen B, Langberg J, Coskun P, Wallace DC, Nesburn AB, Khatibi N, Hertzog D, Le K, Hwang D, Kenney MC: Mitochondrial DNA haplogroups associated with age-related macular degeneration. Invest Ophthalmol Vis Sci 2009; 50:2966–2974.
99 San Giovanni JP, Arking DE, Iyengar SK, Elashoff M, Clemons TE, Reed GF, Henning AK, Sivakumaran TA, Xu X, De Wan A, Agron E, Rochtchina E, Sue CM, Wang JJ, Mitchell P, Hoh J, Francis PJ, Klein ML, Chew EY, Chakravarti A: Mitochondrial DNA variants of respiratory complex I that uniquely characterize haplogroup t2 are associated with increased risk of age-related macular degeneration. PLoS ONE 2009;4: e5508.
100 Kanda A, Chen W, Othman M, Branham KE, Brooks M, Khanna R, He S, Lyons R, Abecasis GR, Swaroop A: A variant of mitochondrial protein LOC387715/ARMS2, not HTRA1, is strongly associated with age-related macular degeneration. Proc Natl Acad SciUSA 2007;104:16227–16232.
101 Fritsche LG, Loenhardt T, Janssen A, Fisher SA, Rivera A, Keilhauer CN, Weber BH: Age-related macular degeneration is associated with an unstable ARMS2 (LOC387715) mRNA. Nat Genet 2008;40: 892–896.
102 Kortvely E, Hauck SM, Duetsch G, Gloeckner CJ, Kremmer E, Alge-Priglinger CS, Deeg C, Ueffing M: ARMS2 is a constituent of the extracellular matrix providing a link between familial and sporadic age-related macular degenerations. Invest Ophthalmol Vis Sci 20010;51:79–88.
103 Barreau E, Brossas JY, Courtois Y, Treton JA: Accumulation of mitochondrial DNA deletions in human retina during aging. Invest Ophthalmol Vis Sci 1996;37:384–391.
104 Wang AL, Lukas TJ, Yuan M, Neufeld AH: Increased mitochondrial DNA damage and down-regulation of DNA repair enzymes in aged rodent retinal pigment epithelium and choroid. Mol Vis 2008;14:644–651.
105 Godley BF, Xu H, Havey A, Xhong X, Lin H, Boulton ME: Mitochondrial DNA repair capacity decreases with progression of age-related macular degeneration (ARVO E-abstract). Invest Ophthalmol Vis Sci 2008; 49.
106 Liang FQ, Godley BF: Oxidative stress-induced mitochondrial DNA damage in human retinal pigment epithelial cells: a possible mechanism for RPE aging and age-related macular degeneration. Exp Eye Res 2003;76:397–403.
107 Nordgaard CL, Berg KM, Kapphahn RJ, Reilly C, Feng X, Olsen TW, Ferrington DA: Proteomics of the retinal pigment epithelium reveals altered protein expression at progressive stages of age-related macular degeneration. Invest Ophthalmol Vis Sci 2006;47:815–822.
108 Nordgaard CL, Karunadharma PP, Feng X, Olsen TW, Ferrington DA: Mitochondrial proteomics of the retinal pigment epithelium at progressive stages of age-related macular degeneration. Invest Ophthalmol Vis Sci 2008;49:2848–2855.
109 Decanini A, Nordgaard CL, Feng X, Ferrington DA, Olsen TW: Changes in select redox proteins of the retinal pigment epithelium in age-related macular degeneration. Am J Ophthalmol 2007;143:607–615.
110 Justilien V, Pang JJ, Renganathan K, Zhan X, Crabb JW, Kim SR, Sparrow JR, Hauswirth WW, Lewin AS: Sod2 knockdown mouse model of early AMD. Invest Ophthalmol Vis Sci 2007;48:4407–4420.
111 Jarrett SG, Boulton ME: Antioxidant up-regulation and increased nuclear DNA protection play key roles in adaptation to oxidative stress in epithelial cells. Free Radic Biol Med 2005;38:1382–1391.
112 Ballinger SW, Van Houten B, Jin GF, Conklin CA, Godley BF: Hydrogen peroxide causes significant mitochondrial DNA damage in human RPE cells. Exp Eye Res 1999;68:765–772.
113 Bosch-Morell F, Roma J, Marin N, Romero B, Rodriguez-Galietero A, Johnsen-Soriano S, Diaz-Llopis M, Romero FJ: Role of oxygen and nitrogen species in experimental uveitis: anti-inflammatory activity of the synthetic antioxidant ebselen. Free Radic Biol Med 2002;33:669–675.
114 Rajendram R, Saraswathy S, Rao NA: Photoreceptor mitochondrial oxidative stress in early experimental autoimmune uveoretinitis. Br J Ophthalmol 2007;91:531–537.
115 Saraswathy S, Rao NA: Mitochondrial proteomics in experimental autoimmune uveitis oxidative stress. Invest Ophthalmol Vis Sci 2009;50:5559–5566.

116 Kong GY, Van Bergen NJ, Trounce IA, Crowston JG: Mitochondrial dysfunction and glaucoma. J Glaucoma 2009;18:93–100.
117 Simpkins JW, Wang J, Wang X, Perez E, Prokai L, Dykens JA: Mitochondria play a central role in estrogen-induced neuroprotection. Curr Drug Targets 2005;4:69–83.
118 Tezel G: Oxidative stress in glaucomatous neurodegeneration:mechanisms and consequences. Prog Retin Eye Res 2006;25:490–513.
119 Osborne NN, Lascaratos G, Bron AJ, Chidlow G, Wood JP: A hypothesis to suggest that light is a risk factor in glaucoma and the mitochondrial optic neuropathies. Br J Ophthalmol 2006;90:237–241.
120 Lascaratos G, Ji D, Wood JP, Osborne NN: Visible light affects mitochondrial function and induces neuronal death in retinal cell cultures. Vis Res 2007;47:1191–1201.
121 Tatton WG, Chalmers-Redman RM, Sud A, Podos SM, Mittag TW: Maintaining mitochondrial membrane impermeability: an opportunity for new therapy in glaucoma? Surv Ophthalmol 2001;45(suppl 3):S277–S283, discussion S295–S296.
122 Mittag TW, Danias J, Pohorenec G, Yuan HM, Burakgazi E, Chalmers-Redman R, Podos SM, Tatton WG: Retinal damage after 3 to 4 months of elevated intraocular pressure in a rat glaucoma model. Invest Ophthalmol Vis Sci 2000;41:3451–3459.
123 Abu-Amero KK, Morales J, Bosley TM: Mitochondrial abnormalities in patients with primary open-angle glaucoma. Invest Ophthalmol Vis Sci 2006;47:2533–2541.
124 Kanwar M, Chan PS, Kern TS, Kowluru RA: Oxidative damage in the retinal mitochondria of diabetic mice: possible protection by superoxide dismutase. Invest Ophthalmol Vis Sci 2007;48:3805–3811.
125 Kowluru RA, Abbas SN: Diabetes-induced mitochondrial dysfunction in the retina. Invest Ophthalmol Vis Sci 2003;44:5327–5334.
126 Ellis EA, Guberski DL, Somogyi-Mann M, Grant MB: Increased H_2O_2, vascular endothelial growth factor and receptors in the retina of the BBZ/WOR diabetic rat. Free Radic Biol Med 2000;28:91–101.
127 Kowluru RA, Chan PS: Oxidative stress and diabetic retinopathy. Exp Diabetes Res 2007;2007:43603.
128 Lin Y, Berg AH, Iyengar P, Lam TK, Giacca A, Combs TP, Rajala MW, Du X, Rollman B, Li W, Hawkins M, Barzilai N, Rhodes CJ, Fantus IG, Brownlee M, Scherer PE: The hyperglycemia-induced inflammatory response in adipocytes: the role of reactive oxygen species. J Biol Chem 2005;280:4617–4626.
129 Santos DL, Palmeira CM, Seica R, Dias J, Mesquita J, Moreno AJ, Santos MS: Diabetes and mitochondrial oxidative stress:a study using heart mitochondria from the diabetic Goto-Kakizaki rat. Mol Cell Biochem 2003;246:163–170.
130 Yorek MA: The role of oxidative stress in diabetic vascular and neural disease. Free Radic Res 2003;37:471–480.
131 Busik JV, Mohr S, Grant MB: Hyperglycemia-induced reactive oxygen species toxicity to endothelial cells is dependent on paracrine mediators. Diabetes 2008;57:1952–1965.
132 Nishikawa T, Kukidome D, Sonoda K, Fujisawa K, Matsuhisa T, Motoshima H, Matsumura T, Araki E: Impact of mitochondrial ROS production on diabetic vascular complications. Diabetes Res Clin Pract 2007;77(suppl 1):S41–S45.
133 Kowluru RA, Atasi L, Ho YS: Role of mitochondrial superoxide dismutase in the development of diabetic retinopathy. Invest Ophthalmol Vis Sci 2006;47:1594–1599.
134 Kowluru RA, Kowluru V, Xiong Y, Ho YS: Overexpression of mitochondrial superoxide dismutase in mice protects the retina from diabetes-induced oxidative stress. Free Radic Biol Med 2006;41:1191–1196.
135 Kowluru RA: Effect of reinstitution of good glycemic control on retinal oxidative stress and nitrative stress in diabetic rats. Diabetes 2003;52:818–823.
136 Stitt AW, Curtis TM: Advanced glycation and retinal pathology during diabetes. Pharmacol Rep 2005;57(suppl):156–168.
137 Uchigata Y, Okada T, Gong JS, Yamada Y, Iwamoto Y, Tanaka M: A mitochondrial genotype associated with the development of autoimmune-related type 1 diabetes. Diabetes Care 2002;25:2106.
138 Mathews CE, Leiter EH, Spirina O, Bykhovskaya Y, Gusdon AM, Ringquist S, Fischel-Ghodsian N: MT-ND2 allele of the ALR/LT mouse confers resistance against both chemically induced and autoimmune diabetes. Diabetologia 2005;48:261–267.
139 Gusdon AM, Votyakova TV, Mathews CE: MT-ND2a suppresses reactive oxygen species production by mitochondrial complexes i and III. J Biol Chem 2008;283:10690–10697.
140 Lou MF: Redox regulation in the lens. Prog Retinal Eye Res 2003;22:657–682.
141 Huang L, Tang D, Yappert MC, Borchman D: Oxidation-induced changes in human lens epithelial cells. 2. Mitochondria and the generation of reactive oxygen species. Free Radic Biol Med 2006;41:926–936.
142 Spector A: Oxidative stress-induced cataract: mechanism of action. Faseb J 1995;9:1173–1182.
143 Yao K, Zhang L, Ye PP, Tang XJ, Zhang YD: Protective effect of magnolol against hydrogen peroxide-induced oxidative stress in human lens epithelial cells. Am J Chin Med 2009;37:785–796.
144 Hightower KR, Duncan G, Dawson A, Wormstone IM, Reddan J, Dziedizc D: Ultraviolet irradiation (UVB) interrupts calcium cell signaling in lens epithelial cells. Photochem Photobiol 1999;69:595–598.
145 Reddan JR, Giblin FJ, Kadry R, Leverenz VR, Pena JT, Dziedzic DC: Protection from oxidative insult in glutathione depleted lens epithelial cells. Exp Eye Res 1999;68:117–127.
146 Di Fonzo A, Ronchi D, Lodi T, Fassone E, Tigano M, Lamperti C, Corti S, Bordoni A, Fortunato F, Nizzardo M, Napoli L, Donadoni C, Salani S, Saladino F, Moggio M, Bresolin N, Ferrero I, Comi GP: The mitochondrial disulfide relay system protein GFER is mutated in autosomal-recessive myopathy with cataract and combined respiratory-chain deficiency. Am J Hum Genet 2009;84:594–604.

Ophthalmic Research

Ophthalmic Res 2010;44:191–198
DOI: 10.1159/000316476

Received: January 27, 2010
Accepted after revision: March 22, 2010
Published online: September 9, 2010

Free Radicals, Antioxidants and Eye Diseases: Evidence from Epidemiological Studies on Cataract and Age-Related Macular Degeneration

A.E. Fletcher

Department of Epidemiology and Population Health, London School of Hygiene and Tropical Medicine, London, UK

Key Words

Free radicals · Age-related cataract · Age-related macular degeneration

Abstract

Cataract and age-related macular degeneration (AMD) are the major causes of vision impairment and blindness worldwide. Both conditions are strongly age related with earlier signs (usually asymptomatic) occurring in middle age and becoming severer and more prevalent with increasing age. The aetiology of these conditions is thought to fit with the 'free radical theory' of ageing which postulates that ageing and age-related diseases result from the accumulation of cellular damage from reactive oxygen species (ROS). Mitochondrial energy production is a major source of endogenous ROS. External sources of ROS include environmental sources especially solar radiation, biomass fuels and tobacco smoking. There is strong evidence from epidemiological studies that smoking is a risk factor for both cataract and AMD. There is moderate evidence for an association with sunlight and cataract but weak evidence for sunlight and AMD. The few studies that have investigated this suggest an adverse effect of biomass fuels on cataract risk. The antioxidant defence system of the lens and retina include antioxidant vitamins C and E and the carotenoids lutein and zinc, and there is mixed evidence on their associations with cataract and AMD from epidemiological studies. Most epidemiological studies have been conducted in well-nourished western populations but evidence is now emerging from other populations with different dietary patterns and antioxidant levels.

Introduction

Cataract and age-related macular degeneration (AMD) are the major causes of vision impairment and blindness worldwide and occur almost exclusively in the older population [1]. AMD and cataract are typical age-related conditions. The prevalence is low in middle age and rises with advancing age. AMD and cataract are not found at younger ages (other than for rare genetic types or due to environmental insults such as trauma or extreme light exposure); earlier, usually asymptomatic, signs of the conditions are, however, found in middle age or earlier in late life, and both the prevalence of these earlier signs and their severity increases with advancing age. A pooled analysis of the major population-based studies in developed country settings (mainly the USA) described prevalence rates of significant lens opacities ranging from

KARGER

Fax +41 61 306 12 34
E-Mail karger@karger.ch
www.karger.com

0030–3747/10/0443–0191$26.00/0

Accessible online at:
www.karger.com/ore

A.E. Fletcher
Department of Epidemiology and Population Health
London School of Hygiene and Tropical Medicine
Keppel Street, London WC1E 7HT (UK)
Tel. +44 207 927 2253/4, Fax +44 207 580 6897, E-Mail astrid.fletcher@lshtm.ac.uk

around 2% at ages 40–49, 15% at ages 60–64 up to over 50% of those aged 75 [2]. In low-income countries, the prevalence of significant lens opacities is much higher than at comparable ages in developed country settings, a finding which does not appear to be explained solely by better access to cataract surgery [3] and may give clues to environmental or genetic factors. AMD also shows a similar pattern with asymptomatic retinal changes being more prevalent in late middle age while the prevalence of late AMD (subtypes choroidal neovascularization and geographic atrophy) rises exponentially with advancing age from the sixth decade. Studies have shown that by ages 65–69, up to half of men and women in the population have drusen and/or pigmentary irregularities [4–6]. The prevalence of late AMD is of the order of 3–5% in the population aged over 65 years, rising to around 20% in people aged 85 years and over [4, 7].

The aetiology of AMD and cataract can be seen within the framework of ageing and age-related conditions considered to result from the lifelong accumulation of molecular damage, in particular from reactive oxygen species (ROS). In the retina, manifestations of ROS damage – lipofuscin accumulation, drusen formation and damage to Bruch's membrane – are considered to be critical factors in the development of AMD [9] while in the lens ROS damage to the lens includes oxidation of α-crystallin protein disrupting the refractive index, light scattering and loss of transparency [10]. In addition to oxidative stress, advanced glycation end products accumulate with age and are more common in ageing cells, such as the nuclear fibres, drusen and Bruch's membrane, in people with diabetes and in smokers [11].

Endogenous Sources of ROS – The Importance of Mitochondria

Over 50 years ago, Harman [12] proposed that endogenous free radical damage led to the degenerative changes associated with ageing and some 20 years later further hypothesized that mitochondrial energy production was the major source of cellular free radicals [13]. Evidence from numerous subsequent studies has confirmed the importance of mitochondrial respiration [14] with estimates that up to 90% of cellular ROS originate in the mitochondria [15]. Further evidence for the role of mitochondria in ageing include the elucidation of the mitochondrial antioxidant defence system, the age-related accumulation of mitochondrial damage from ROS including increased generation of ROS, mitochondrial apoptosis and deletions in mitochondrial DNA (mtDNA).

Much of the research on mitochondrial function and mtDNA variants has been undertaken in laboratory animals using measures of ageing or specific organs, in particular the brain [16], and studies of Parkinson's disease and Alzheimer's disease [17], and only recently have studies on mitochondrial function in age-related eye disease emerged [18, 19] with several studies describing associations with AMD and variants in mtDNA independent of associations with variants in the nuclear genome [20–22].

Caloric restriction has been proposed as a method to decrease mitochondrial ROS generation. Much of the evidence is based on carefully controlled experiments with laboratory animals including primates and studies from highly selected groups of human volunteers although the first results from randomized controlled trials (RCTs) are emerging [23]. No study has investigated the effects of caloric restriction on cataract or AMD or any other age-related eye conditions. However, since cataracts are more prevalent in populations characterized by indices of poor nutrition including anthropometric measures (low body mass index) [24] or low levels of antioxidant vitamins [25], it is clear that caloric restriction must be considered in the context of the overall nutritional quality of the diet. Conversely, there is some evidence from well-nourished western populations that indicators of excess caloric consumption such as obesity are associated with cataract [26] and AMD [27] although whether these associations are independent of the association with diabetes remains unclear.

Exogenous Sources of ROS

Exogenous sources include environmental factors such as solar radiation, particulates (e.g. from burning fossil fuels or biomass fuels) or tobacco. The eye is particularly exposed to the damaging effects of light. Visible light consists of wavelengths between 400 and 700 nm corresponding to colour ranges from violet/blue light (shortest wavelengths) to orange and red. Ultraviolet light radiation (UVR), not visible to the human eye, covers a range of shorter wavelengths beyond 400 nm and consists of UVA (315–400 nm), UVB (280–315 nm) and UVC (less than 280 nm). The shorter wavelengths of light have the highest energy compared to longer wavelengths and hence the greatest potential for adverse effects, e.g. by ROS generation. All UVC and around 90% of UVB light is absorbed by the ozone layer. The retina is protected against UVR by the cornea and the lens, which absorbs wavelengths below 370 nm increasing to up to 470 nm as the lens yellows with age, and opacities, especially nuclear opacities, are formed [28].

The lens and retina contain a number of potent antioxidants, some at very high concentrations compared to elsewhere in the body. These include glutathione and related enzymes, principally glutathione reductase and glutathione peroxidase. Others include superoxide dismutase and catalase, antioxidant vitamins like vitamin C, E and the carotenoids (carotene, lutein and zeaxanthin) and minerals such as selenium (lens) and zinc (retina) [9]. The antioxidant enzymes are the first-line defence system supported by the antioxidant vitamins. Vitamin C (ascorbate) is the most important antioxidant vitamin in the lens and found in the aqueous at concentrations of 30- to 50-fold that of the plasma [29]. Vitamin E is found in the lens but at similar levels to those in the plasma. Vitamin C acts synergistically with vitamin E, and both vitamins C and E maintain the antioxidant activity of glutathione [30]. Lutein and zeaxanthin are the main lens carotenoids; very little β-carotene is present [31]. The only carotenoids found in the retina are lutein and zeaxanthin which are present in very high concentrations in the macula. These carotenoids scavenge singlet oxygen (one of the most damaging ROS) and also protect the cell membranes from lipid oxidation. In addition they filter harmful blue light [32]. Zinc is found in high concentrations in photoreceptors and RPE cells. These antioxidants cannot be synthesized by the body and must be obtained from dietary sources.

Epidemiological Evidence on Exogenous Oxidative Stress

Light Exposure

Few studies have investigated associations of solar radiation and lens opacities or AMD in human populations, perhaps because of the challenges of measurement of long-term exposures. Exposure to sunlight has been related to cortical cataracts in some studies but not observed in all [33]. Two studies have reported an association with nuclear cataract [34, 35] but this was not found in other studies. Similarly, the evidence has been inconsistent for AMD. A study of fishermen found an association with estimated 20-year exposure to blue light and risk of geographic atrophy [36]. The Beaver Dam and POLA studies estimated potential maximum UVR exposure [37, 38] based on residence but did not take account of the actual time spent outdoors or the use of ocular protection. Neither study found an association with UVR and AMD while the POLA study found a reduced association of increasing UVR with early AMD [38]. Other studies based only on self-reports of time spent outdoors found either no association [39–41] or that leisure time outdoors in young adult life was associated with early, but not late, AMD [42]. All previous studies examined only the effects of sunlight exposure and did not take account of other factors such as diet although it is plausible that the adverse effects of sunlight are modified by diet, specifically antioxidants. The EUREYE study investigated this hypothesis [8]. Blue light exposure was estimated from meteorological data based on lifetime residence and information on terrain and cloud cover. Information from the questionnaire on outdoor exposure and the use of ocular protection during different life periods was used to estimate the proportion of maximum exposure actually experienced by an individual. The results showed a significant adverse association of blue light exposure on the risk of late AMD (choroidal neovascularization) in those with the lowest antioxidant levels (defined as those in the lowest quarter) of vitamin C, zeaxanthin, vitamin E and dietary zinc with an odds ratio (OR) of about 1.4 for 1 standard deviation unit increase in blue light exposure (fig. 1). Higher ORs (around 4-fold) for blue light

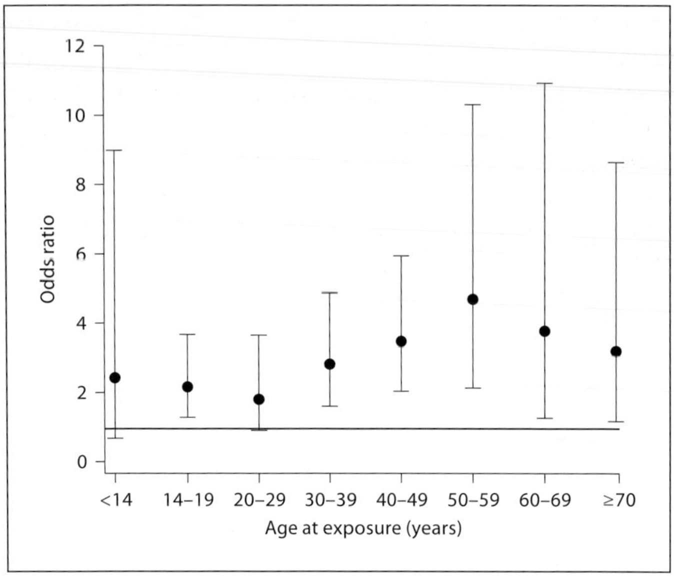

Fig. 1. Association of mean annual midday blue light exposure with neovascular AMD by age at exposure in those with lowest joint quartiles of vitamin C, zeaxanthin and vitamin E: odds ratios with 95% confidence intervals (expressed as vertical bars). From Fletcher et al. [8].

Table 1. Association of midday blue light exposure with neovascular AMD by joint low levels of antioxidants

Joint lowest quartile of antioxidants	OR	95% CI	p value[1]	p value[2]
Vitamin C and zeaxanthin	1.66	1.15–2.38	0.02	0.05
Vitamin C and lutein	1.37	0.60–3.09	0.4	0.6
Vitamin C and α-tocopherol	2.47	1.65–3.67	0.001	<0.01
Vitamin C and dietary zinc[3]	1.53	1.20–1.95	0.005	0.03
Zeaxanthin and lutein	1.43	0.75–2.73	0.2	0.4
Zeaxanthin and α-tocopherol	2.34	1.61–3.40	0.001	<0.01
Zeaxanthin and dietary zinc[3]	2.60	2.33–2.88	<0.001	<0.001
Lutein and α-tocopherol	1.57	0.64–3.86	0.3	0.4
Vitamin C and zeaxanthin and α-tocopherol	3.72	1.56–8.88	0.01	0.02
Vitamin C and lutein and α-tocopherol	2.61	0.49–13.90	0.2	0.3
Vitamin C and zeaxanthin and dietary zinc[3]	1.97	0.26–1.17	0.1	0.1

From Fletcher et al. [8]. CI = Confidence interval; midday = 11 a.m. to 3 p.m.; joint lowest quartile = combined lowest quartiles. OR was assessed for the effect of 1 SD increase in blue light exposure, adjusted for age, sex, smoking status, diabetes, cardiovascular disease, education, aspirin use, retinol and cholesterol level.

[1] Test of effect of blue light exposure.

[2] Test of interaction between joint lowest quartile of antioxidants with blue light exposure on association with neovascular AMD.

[3] Adjusted for energy intake.

were observed for those who were in the lowest quartile for several antioxidants, such as vitamin C, zeaxanthin and vitamin E (table 1).

Biomass Fuels

Biomass fuels such as wood, crop residues and dried cow dung are common sources of cheap cooking fuel in many low-income countries. The smoke from combustion of these fuels includes small respirable particles, carbon monoxide, nitrogen, formaldehyde and polyaromatic hydrocarbons. The adverse effect of biomass fuels on human health is well documented especially for respiratory conditions [43]. The evidence for eye problems is scanty but suggests that indoor air pollutants may represent a major environmental exposure for cataracts. All studies to date have been conducted in India where biomass fuel use is highly prevalent especially in the rural areas. Two hospital-based case-control studies [44, 45] found increased risks associated with cheap cooking fuels (ORs of 4.13 and 1.6, respectively) while one community-based study [46] in two regional areas found an increased OR (1.8) with use of cheap cooking fuels and cataract, in one area but a reduced association in another. A recent case-control study [47] reported that, compared to clean fuels (biogas, liquefied petroleum gas or kerosene), use of biomass fuel in a stove without a chimney was associated with a 2-fold risk of cataract. Lack of kitchen ventilation was also an independent risk factor for cataract. The plausibility of these associations with biomass fuels is supported by studies in rats showing that smoke condensates prepared from wood smoke result in lens opacification [48] possibly as a result of damage to the lens transport systems leading to an accumulation of smoke metabolites [49]. However, since many of the constituents of biomass fuels are also found in tobacco smoke, it is likely that other adverse effects of biomass fuels on lens opacities are similar to those found for tobacco. Adverse effects of biomass fuels are also likely therefore to affect AMD; however, currently no studies have examined this.

Tobacco Use

Cigarette smoking is a risk factor for most age-related conditions and has been consistently identified as a risk factor for cataract and AMD. That the association is likely to be causal is suggested by the consistency of the association across different study designs and populations, a dose-response relationship and a reduction in risk with length of cessation. A meta-analysis for AMD [50] based on 5 prospective studies and 8 case-control studies reported that current smoking was associated with an approximately 2-fold risk of AMD and past smoking around 1.5. A systematic review of 27 studies of smoking and cataract reported 3-fold incidence rates of nuclear cataract

Table 2. Risk of AMD by category of combined intake of 4 predefined antioxidant nutrients (vitamins C and E, β-carotene and zinc)

	Category of dietary intake		
	low (n = 466)	middle (n = 3,270)	high (n = 434)
Cases of AMD	76 (16.3%)	422 (13.5%)	42 (9.7%)
Hazard ratio			
Unadjusted	1.31 (1.03–1.67)	1.00	0.65 (0.48–0.89)
Age- and sex-adjusted	1.23 (0.97–1.58)	1.00	0.68 (0.49–0.93)
Fully adjusted	1.20 (0.92–1.56)	1.00	0.65 (0.46–0.92)

From van Leeuwen et al. [57]. Ranges in parentheses indicate 95% confidence intervals. Categories were defined by using the median energy-adjusted daily intake as a cutoff value and classifying above-median intake of all nutrients as high intake and below-median intake of all nutrients as low intake. Cutoff values were: 114 mg for vitamin C, 13 mg for vitamin E, 3.6 mg for β-carotene and 9.6 mg for zinc. Fully adjusted = Adjusted for age, sex, body mass index, smoking status, pack-years of smoking, systolic blood pressure, atherosclerosis composite score, serum total cholesterol and alcohol intake.

with smoking [51]. The evidence was less strong for posterior subcapsular or cortical cataract. These studies were based primarily on data from western populations where manufactured cigarettes are the main form of tobacco use. In other populations alternative forms of tobacco include home-grown tobacco such as beedies in India, or tobacco chewing or pipe smoking (hookah). Although the data are sparse, there is some suggestion that beedies confer less or even no risk of cataract. In the Andhra Pradesh Eye Study, western style cigarettes were associated with a 1.5-fold risk of cataract and hookahs with a non-significant 6-fold risk (few hookah smokers in the study) [52]. There was a borderline significantly reduced association of beedie smoking (OR = 0.8). In 2 other studies in India, either no [44] or a weak association [24] was found but these studies did not report the type of cigarettes smoked. Smoking tobacco (92% smoked beedies) was not a risk factor for cataract in a further study [53] but tobacco chewing (common in the south Indian population) was associated with a 1.5-fold increased risk. Beedies contain less tobacco than manufactured cigarettes and combust poorly; it is plausible therefore that beedies have less adverse effects compared to tobacco smoke.

In addition to ROS generation, smoking depletes plasma antioxidant levels [54] and macular pigment (thought to protect against AMD). Both smokers and chewers of tobacco have been shown to exhibit higher levels of cadmium in blood and lens [55]. Cadmium has a range of adverse effects resulting in depleted superoxide dismutase status.

Epidemiological Evidence on Antioxidants

Because of their concentrations and antioxidant activities in the lens and retina, most studies have investigated vitamins C and E and the carotenoids lutein and zeaxanthin. Although the evidence does support a role for antioxidants in the aetiology of AMD and cataract, the evidence for one specific antioxidant over another is inconsistent and only partly accounted for by variations in study design and the methods used to assess antioxidant levels [56]. For the most part, studies have focused on one single antioxidant in exploring associations, although synergistic effects of antioxidants are well known. The few studies that have attempted to construct an overall antioxidant index or examined combinations of the key antioxidants have found inverse associations supporting the overall antioxidant hypothesis; for example, a high dietary intake of β-carotene, vitamins C and E, and zinc was associated with a substantially reduced risk of AMD in elderly persons in the Rotterdam Study [57] (table 2).

Studies have also examined associations between patterns of diet. A higher frequency of intake of spinach or collard greens was associated with a substantially lower risk for neovascular AMD in one study [58]; conversely fruit intake but not vegetables or carotenoids was inversely associated with neovascular AMD in the Health Professionals' and Nurses' Studies [59]. Women in the highest 2 quartiles of a Healthy Eating Index had a 50% reduction in risk of lens opacities; milk, fruit and variety (but not vegetable intake) made the strongest contribution to reduced risk [60]. The overwhelming majority of epidemiological studies have been conducted in well-nourished western populations. In a study in North India, levels of antioxidants (measured in the blood) were lower than reported in western studies, especially vitamin C [25]. Inverse associations were found with a number of antioxidants (including vitamin C, zeaxanthin and retinol) and cataract.

The evidence from high-quality RCTs of supplementation on cataract risk or progression have mainly been negative. No benefit was observed in the AREDS trial for high-dose antioxidant supplements (β-carotene, vitamin C and vitamin E) [61] or the VECAT study using high-dose vitamin E [62]. Supplementation might be expected to have a stronger effect in an antioxidant-depleted population but a trial in southern India found no benefit from supplementation with multivitamins (vitamins A, C and E) on the rate of progression of opacities over a 5-year period [63]. However, a recently published trial in an Italian population using a broad-spectrum multivitamin/mineral supplement found a reduced rate of progression of nuclear opacities and an increased risk of posterior subcapsular opacities [64]. This trial was also of the longest duration (average of 9 years of supplement use). For AMD the strongest evidence of an effect of antioxidant supplementation is provided by the AREDS trial [65], which demonstrated that among people with moderate signs of AMD at baseline taking a high dose of multivitamins (vitamins A, C, E, β-carotene) in combination with zinc was associated with an approximately 25% reduction in 5-year progression. The supplement doses used in the trial were very high, around 10 times of the recommended daily intakes. There is a concern about possible toxicity related to such high doses of antioxidant supplements. A recent meta-analysis of well-conducted randomized trials (47 trials including AREDS, VECAT with 180,938 participants) found an increased mortality risk associated with supplementation beyond the daily recommended doses with a risk estimate of 1.05 (95% confidence interval = 1.02–1.08) [66]. The adverse effect was observed for vitamin A, β-carotene and vitamin E but not for vitamin C.

The lack of clear evidence from RCTs of antioxidant supplementation on a variety of age-related diseases has led to claims that the evidence on antioxidants from observational studies is confounded by other factors associated with healthy diets [67]. However, as argued elsewhere [68], the notion that RCTs of one or even a few supplements over a relatively short period of time can test the evidence on an antioxidant-rich diet is misplaced. First because of the long period of time for the development of late-life diseases and second because the synergy of the full package of dietary antioxidants cannot be replaced with a tablet. Further light on this debate may be provided by the recent identification of genetic variants that influence the blood levels of, and response to, antioxidants [69]. The association of these variants with disease should provide an unconfounded assessment of dietary hypotheses (so-called mendelian randomization).

Variants in a gene affecting vitamin C transport (SLC23A2) were associated with non-Hodgkins lymphoma [70], supporting evidence from epidemiological studies of a lower risk of non-Hodgkins lymphoma in those with higher intakes of fruits and vegetables. Currently the evidence for an association with variants influencing antioxidant levels and disease risk is very limited for cataract and AMD. In a case-control analysis from two populations (France and USA), a weak association between the heterozygote allele of a variant of the SCARB1 gene (rs5888) and AMD was found (OR = 1.4, 95% confidence interval = 1.0–1.8). SCARB1 mediates cholesterol uptake and is involved in the uptake of vitamin E and lutein [71].

Conclusions

Some 60 years since first proposed, there has been a vast amount of work undertaken to elucidate the complex pathways and mechanisms relevant to the free radical theory of ageing. There are considerable challenges in investigating findings from laboratory studies in epidemiological studies in humans. Epidemiological studies are required to provide the evidence supporting public health policies and interventions and to advise the public and patients about the risk or protective factors, especially lifestyle factors, under their control. To date the clearest evidence is the risk of cataract and AMD from smoking. Further understanding of the role of dietary factors, especially with reference to the antioxidant hypothesis, will be provided by studies in diverse populations which are now beginning to emerge.

Conflict of Interest

A.E.F. receives funding from the Wellcome Trust UK for the INDEYE study (a study of risk factors for age-related cataract and AMD in India).

References

1 Resnikoff S, et al: Global data on visual impairment in the year 2002. Bull World Health Organ 2004;82:844–851.

2 Congdon N, et al: Prevalence of cataract and pseudophakia/aphakia among adults in the United States. Arch Ophthalmol 2004;122:487–494.

3 Murthy GV, et al: Prevalence of lens opacities in North India: the INDEYE feasibility study. Invest Ophthalmol Vis Sci 2007;48:88–95.

4 Augood CA, et al: Prevalence of age-related maculopathy in older Europeans: the European Eye Study (EUREYE). Arch Ophthalmol 2006;124:529–535.

5 Klein R, Klein BE, Linton KL: Prevalence of age-related maculopathy. The Beaver Dam Eye Study. Ophthalmology 1992;99:933–943.

6 Vingerling JR, et al: The prevalence of age-related maculopathy in the Rotterdam Study. Ophthalmology 1995;102:205–210.

7 Congdon N, et al: Causes and prevalence of visual impairment among adults in the United States. Arch Opthalmol 2004;122:477–485.

8 Fletcher AE, et al: Sunlight exposure, antioxidants, and age-related macular degeneration. Arch Ophthalmol 2008;126:1396–1403.

9 Winkler BS, et al: Oxidative damage and age-related macular degeneration. Mol Vis 1999;5:32.

10 Berthoud VM, Beyer EC: Oxidative stress, lens gap junctions, and cataracts. Antioxid Redox Signal 2009;11:339–353.

11 Stitt AW: Advanced glycation: an important pathological event in diabetic and age related ocular disease. Br J Ophthalmol 2001;85:746–753.

12 Harman D: Aging: a theory based on free radical and radiation chemistry. J Gerontol 1956;11:298–300.

13 Harman D: The biologic clock: the mitochondria? J Am Geriatr Soc 1972;20:145–147.

14 Muller FL, et al: Trends in oxidative aging theories. Free Radic Biol Med 2007;43:477–503.

15 Balaban RS, Nemoto S, Finkel T: Mitochondria, oxidants, and aging. Cell 2005;120:483–495.

16 Kujoth GC, et al: The role of mitochondrial DNA mutations in mammalian aging. PLoS Genet 2007;3:e24.

17 Beal MF: Mitochondrial dysfunction and oxidative damage in Alzheimer's and Parkinson's diseases and coenzyme Q_{10} as a potential treatment. J Bioenerg Biomembr 2004;36:381–386.

18 Brennan LA, Kantorow M: Mitochondrial function and redox control in the aging eye: role of MsrA and other repair systems in cataract and macular degenerations. Exp Eye Res 2009;88:195–203.

19 Jarrett SG, et al: Mitochondrial DNA damage and its potential role in retinal degeneration. Prog Retinal Eye Res 2008;27:596–607.

20 Canter JA, et al: Mitochondrial DNA polymorphism A4917G is independently associated with age-related macular degeneration. PLoS One 2008;3:e2091.

21 San Giovanni JP, et al: Mitochondrial DNA variants of respiratory complex I that uniquely characterize haplogroup T2 are associated with increased risk of age-related macular degeneration. PLoS One 2009;4:e5508.

22 Udar N, et al: Mitochondrial DNA haplogroups associated with age-related macular degeneration. Invest Ophthalmol Vis Sci 2009;50:2966–2974.

23 Redman LM, et al: Metabolic and behavioral compensations in response to caloric restriction: implications for the maintenance of weight loss. PLoS One 2009;4:e4377.

24 Nirmalan PK, et al: Risk factors for age related cataract in a rural population of southern India: the Aravind Comprehensive Eye Study. Br J Ophthalmol 2004;88:989–994.

25 Dherani M, et al: Blood levels of vitamin C, carotenoids and retinol are inversely associated with cataract in a North Indian population. Invest Ophthalmol Vis Sci 2008;49:3328–3335.

26 Weintraub JM, et al: A prospective study of the relationship between body mass index and cataract extraction among US women and men. Int J Obes Relat Metab Disord 2002;26:1588–1595.

27 Klein R, et al: Cardiovascular disease, its risk factors and treatment, and age-related macular degeneration: Women's Health Initiative Sight Exam ancillary study. Am J Ophthalmol 2007;143:473–483.

28 Oliva MS, Taylor H: Ultraviolet radiation and the eye. Int Ophthalmol Clin 2005;45:1–17.

29 Varma SD: Ascorbic acid and the eye with special reference to the lens. Ann NY Acad Sci 1987;498:280–306.

30 Shang F, et al: Vitamin C and vitamin E restore the resistance of GSH-depleted lens cells to H_2O_2. Free Radic Biol Med 2003;34:521–530.

31 Taylor A, Hobbs M: 2001 assessment of nutritional influences on risk for cataract. Nutrition 2001;17:845–857.

32 Beatty S, et al: Macular pigment and age related macular degeneration. Br J Ophthalmol 1999;83:867–877.

33 McCarty CA, Taylor HR: A review of the epidemiologic evidence linking ultraviolet radiation and cataracts. Dev Ophthalmol 2002;35:21–31.

34 Neale RE, et al: Sun exposure as a risk factor for nuclear cataract. Epidemiology 2003;14:707–712.

35 Pastor-Valero M, et al: Years of sunlight exposure and cataract: a case-control study in a Mediterranean population. BMC Ophthalmol 2007;7:18.

36 Taylor HR, et al: The long-term effects of visible light on the eye. Arch Ophthalmol 1992;110:99–104.

37 Cruickshanks KJ, Klein R, Klein BE: Sunlight and age-related macular degeneration. The Beaver Dam Eye Study. Arch Ophthalmol 1993;111:514–518.

38 Delcourt C, et al: Light exposure and the risk of age-related macular degeneration: the Pathologies Oculaires Liéés à l'Age (POLA) study. Arch Ophthalmol 2001;119:1463–1468.

39 Darzins P, Mitchell P, Heller RF: Sun exposure and age-related macular degeneration: an Australian case-control study. Ophthalmology 1997;104:770–776.

40 The Eye Disease Case-Control Study Group: Risk factors for neovascular age-related macular degeneration. Arch Ophthalmol 1992;110:1701–1708.

41 Khan JC, et al: Age related macular degeneration and sun exposure, iris colour, and skin sensitivity to sunlight. Br J Ophthalmol 2006;90:29–32.

42 Cruickshanks KJ, et al: Sunlight and the 5-year incidence of early age-related maculopathy: the Beaver Dam Eye Study. Arch Ophthalmol 2001;119:246–250.

43 Bruce N, Perez-Padilla R, Albalak R: Indoor air pollution in developing countries: a major environmental and public health challenge. Bull World Health Organ 2000;78:1078–1092.

44 Mohan M, et al: India-US case-control study of age-related cataracts. India-US Case-Control Study Group. Arch Ophthalmol 1989;107:670–676.

45 Ughade SN, Zodpey SP, Khanolkar VA: Risk factors for cataract: a case control study. Indian J Ophthalmol 1998;46:221–227.

46 Sreenivas V, et al: A rural population based case-control study of senile cataract in India. J Epidemiol 1999;9:327–336.

47 Pokhrel AK, et al: Case-control study of indoor cooking smoke exposure and cataract in Nepal and India. Int J Epidemiol 2005;34:702–708.

48 Shalini VK, et al: Oxidative damage to the eye lens caused by cigarette smoke and fuel smoke condensates. Indian J Biochem Biophys 1994;31:261–266.

49 Rao CM, et al: Effect of smoke condensate on the physiological integrity and morphology of organ cultured rat lenses. Curr Eye Res 1995;14:295–301.

50 Cong R, et al: Smoking and the risk of age-related macular degeneration: a meta-analysis. Ann Epidemiol 2008;18:647–656.

51 Kelly SP, et al: Smoking and cataract: review of causal association. J Cataract Refract Surg 2005;31:2395–2404.

52 Krishnaiah S, et al: Smoking and its association with cataract: results of the Andhra Pradesh eye disease study from India. Invest Ophthalmol Vis Sci 2005;46:58–65.
53 Raju P, et al: Influence of tobacco use on cataract development. Br J Ophthalmol 2006; 90:1374–1377.
54 Dietrich M, et al: Smoking and exposure to environmental tobacco smoke decrease some plasma antioxidants and increase γ-tocopherol in vivo after adjustment for dietary antioxidant intakes. Am J Clin Nutr 2003;77:160–166.
55 Ramakrishnan S, et al: Smoking of beedies and cataract: cadmium and vitamin C in the lens and blood. Br J Ophthalmol 1995;79: 202–206.
56 Chiu CJ, Taylor A: Nutritional antioxidants and age-related cataract and maculopathy. Exp Eye Res 2007;84:229–245.
57 Van Leeuwen R, et al: Dietary intake of antioxidants and risk of age-related macular degeneration. JAMA 2005;294:3101–3107.
58 Seddon JM, et al: Dietary carotenoids, vitamins A, C, and E, and advanced age-related macular degeneration. Eye Disease Case-Control Study Group. JAMA 1994;272:1413–1420.
59 Cho E, et al: Prospective study of intake of fruits, vegetables, vitamins, and carotenoids and risk of age-related maculopathy. Arch Ophthalmol 2004;122:883–892.
60 Moeller SM, et al: Overall adherence to the dietary guidelines for Americans is associated with reduced prevalence of early age-related nuclear lens opacities in women. J Nutr 2004;134:1812–1819.
61 A randomized, placebo-controlled, clinical trial of high-dose supplementation with vitamins C and E and beta carotene for age-related cataract and vision loss: AREDS report No 9. Arch Ophthalmol 2001;119: 1439–1452.
62 McNeil JJ, et al: Vitamin E supplementation and cataract: randomized controlled trial. Ophthalmology 2004;111:75–84.
63 Gritz DC, et al: The Antioxidants in Prevention of Cataracts Study: effects of antioxidant supplements on cataract progression in South India. Br J Ophthalmol 2006;90:847–851.
64 Maraini G, et al: A randomized, double-masked, placebo-controlled clinical trial of multivitamin supplementation for age-related lens opacities. Clinical trial of nutritional supplements and age-related cataract report No 3. Ophthalmology 2008;115:599–607 e1.
65 A randomized, placebo-controlled, clinical trial of high-dose supplementation with vitamins C and E, beta carotene, and zinc for age-related macular degeneration and vision loss: AREDS report No 8. Arch Ophthalmol 2001;119:1417–1436.
66 Bjelakovic G, et al: Antioxidant supplements for prevention of mortality in healthy participants and patients with various diseases. Cochrane Database Syst Rev 2008;CD007176.
67 Lawlor DA, et al: Those confounded vitamins: what can we learn from the differences between observational versus randomised trial evidence? Lancet 2004;363:1724–1727.
68 Fletcher AE: Controversy over 'contradiction': should randomized trials always trump observational studies? Am J Ophthalmol 2009;147:384–386.
69 Loktionov A: Common gene polymorphisms and nutrition: emerging links with pathogenesis of multifactorial chronic diseases (review). J Nutr Biochem 2003;14:426–451.
70 Skibola CF, et al: Polymorphisms in the estrogen receptor 1 and vitamin C and matrix metalloproteinase gene families are associated with susceptibility to lymphoma. PLoS One 2008;3:e2816.
71 Zerbib J, et al: rs5888 variant of SCARB1 gene is a possible susceptibility factor for age-related macular degeneration. PLoS One 2009;4:e7341.

Ophthalmic Research

Ophthalmic Res 2010;44:199–203
DOI: 10.1159/000316484

Published online: September 9, 2010

Retinal Aging and Sirtuins

Yoko Ozawa[a, b] Shunsuke Kubota[a, b] Toshio Narimatsu[a, b] Kenya Yuki[a, b]
Takashi Koto[a, b] Mariko Sasaki[a, b] Kazuo Tsubota[b]

[a] Laboratory of Retinal Cell Biology and [b] Department of Ophthalmology, Keio University School of Medicine, Tokyo, Japan

Key Words
Cell senescence · Apoptosis · Retinal aging · Sirtuin

Abstract
The process of aging involves the accumulating changes in the microenvironment that lead to cell senescence or apoptosis, and subsequent tissue or organ dysfunction. Multiple extrinsic and intrinsic events that cause DNA instability are associated with aging. Cells containing unstable DNA are biologically vulnerable, and if the DNA damage is too great for the cell to repair, it becomes senescent or dies by apoptosis. Thus, the cell's capacity to repair its DNA determines the progress of aging, at least in part. Here, we focus on the sirtuins, the mammalian homologs of the yeast life-span-extending molecule, Sir2. Among the sirtuin family proteins in mammals, the one most similar to yeast Sir2 is SIRT1, which is involved in multiple pathways, including the repair of DNA double-strand breaks. Although the role of SIRT1 in mammalian longevity is not clear, it is expressed throughout the retina, where it may suppress aging. In fact, a mutant mouse model of retinal degeneration shows an abnormal subcellular localization of SIRT1 protein and accelerated retinal cell apoptosis. Further analyses are required to elucidate the mechanism of DNA damage and repair, including the contributions of the sirtuins, in the aged or diseased retinas, which will help us understand the mechanisms of retinal aging.

Accumulating changes in the microenvironment promote the aging of tissues and organs, which can eventually lead to their malfunction. The underlying mechanisms have long been explored, and their molecular basis is beginning to emerge. In this section, we describe how aging is evaluated scientifically and why sirtuins are an important topic in aging science. We also discuss the possible role of sirtuins in retinal aging.

Aging of a Tissue/Organ and DNA Instability

Aging research attracts the attention of researchers across various biological fields. Not only the length of the individual life span, but also the duration of tissue or organ function is of interest. In skin biology, the mechanism of 'photoaging', through which skin aging is accelerated by light exposure, has been widely investigated [1]. UV irradiation results in DNA damage in skin cells, which triggers DNA damage responses, including DNA repair. However, when the damage exceeds the ability of the cell to repair it, a cell cycle checkpoint response is triggered that leads to growth arrest and premature senescence, or to apoptosis, in order to prevent the genomic abnormality and instability from being inherited by other cells. In this case, aging is induced through an extrinsic mechanism.

On the other hand, telomeres, protective DNA structures at the ends of the chromosomes, are progressively

KARGER

Fax +41 61 306 12 34
E-Mail karger@karger.ch
www.karger.com

0030–3747/10/0443–0199$26.00/0

Accessible online at:
www.karger.com/ore

Yoko Ozawa, MD, PhD
Department of Ophthalmology, Keio University School of Medicine
35 Shinanomachi
Shinjuku-ku, Tokyo 160-8582 (Japan)
Tel. +81 3 3353 1211, Fax +81 3 3359 8302, E-Mail yoko-o@sc.itc.keio.ac.jp

shortened during cell division, because the DNA replication machineries incompletely copy the 3′ DNA ends, thereby inducing DNA loss [2]. Finally, this intrinsic mechanism causes the telomeres to shorten beyond a critical point that elicits a DNA damage response. This response causes irreversible cell cycle arrest (senescence), in cells that originally had normal genetic information.

Therefore, excessive DNA instability, induced by extrinsic or intrinsic events, to a level beyond its ability to be repaired, causes cell cycle arrest or apoptosis. As the number of senescent cells increases and that of normal-functioning cells decreases, the tissue/organ becomes compromised and aged.

The retina is part of the central nervous system, and mature retinal cells are thought never to divide under normal conditions. Thus, cell cycle withdrawal occurs physiologically. Most neuronal cells in the brain do not proliferate either. Thus, decreases in functioning cells in the central nervous system may more easily lead to tissue/organ dysfunction and aging than in other parts of the body [3, 4]. Abnormal DNA is a pathological finding associated with some age-related neurodegenerative diseases, consistent with our understanding of aging as a consequence of DNA instability.

Various cytokines may also play a role in the aging process, again as a result of DNA instability [2]. In senescent human fibroblasts and epithelial cells, more than 40 distinct molecules can be secreted in response to DNA damage. Thus, chronic, not transient, changes in the microenvironment, due to the secretion of cytokines such as interleukins 6 or 8, may be induced by DNA instability during tissue/organ aging.

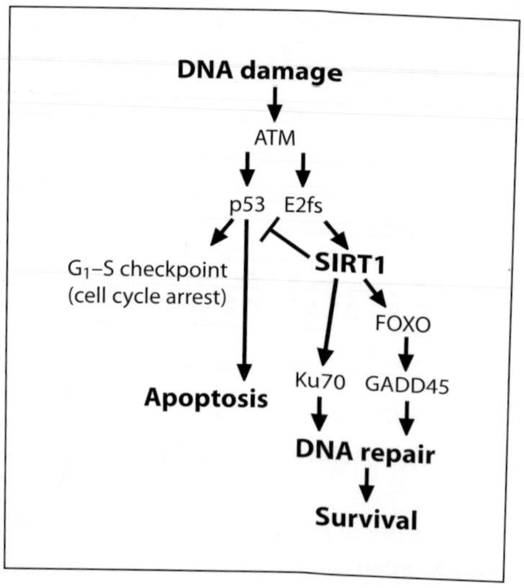

Fig. 1. SIRT1 in the DNA damage response. DNA damage (double-strand breaks) induces ataxia telangiectasia mutated (ATM), which activates p53 to slow the cell cycle (cell cycle checkpoints) to gain time for DNA repair. ATM also activates SIRT1 through E2fs, which in turn activates Ku70 (a protein for double-strand break repair), for the purpose of DNA repair and cell survival, and suppresses p53, to inhibit apoptosis. SIRT1 can also associate with forkhead transcription factor (FOXO) to induce antiapoptotic factors, such as manganese superoxide dismutase and growth-arrest- and DNA-damage-inducible protein 45 (GADD45, a protein for DNA repair).

DNA Instability and Sirtuins

Once DNA damage occurs, it triggers a series of downstream events, the purpose of which is to maintain and promote the survival of the tissue/organ as a whole [5, 6]. First, cell proliferation is interrupted to allow time for DNA repair before synthesis. Then, if the repair is unsuccessful, processes to eliminate the cells are initiated.

Among the types of DNA damage, which include DNA single-strand breaks and base damage, DNA double-strand breaks are the hardest to repair, since both alleles are damaged simultaneously, leaving no complete template for the repair. In one of the main repair systems for double-strand breaks, nonhomologous end-joining, a serine/threonine-specific protein kinase, ataxia telangiectasia mutated (ATM), is induced and activates p53 to stop the cell cycle at the G_1 phase, preventing it from entering the S phase (fig. 1). Such a pause in cell cycle progression is termed a 'cell cycle checkpoint'. ATM activates the E2f transcription factors, which upregulate SIRT1. Deacetylation by SIRT1 activates Ku70, a nonhomologous end-joining DNA repair protein, while SIRT1 activity inhibits excessive activation of p53 and apoptosis. Therefore, SIRT1 regulates DNA stability and promotes cell survival.

SIRT1 is a mammalian homolog of yeast silent information regulator (Sir) 2, which plays a role in the life span extension by caloric restriction in yeast [7, 8]. Sirtuins are class III histone deacetylases, which require nicotinamide adenine dinucleotide (NAD) as a cofactor. There are 7 mammalian Sir2 family members, designated SIRT1–SIRT7 [3, 9–12] (table 1), with SIRT1 being the most highly related to yeast Sir2 [3, 9, 13, 14]. The contribution of SIRT1/Sir2 to genome stability was shown in yeast cells and mouse embryonic stem cells [4]. SIRT1,

Table 1. Mammalian sirtuins

Human sirtuin	Subcellular localization	Enzyme activity	Biology
SIRT1	Nucleus (cytosol)	Deacetylase	DNA stability and cell proliferation (DNA double-strand break repair)
SIRT2	Cytosol	Deacetylase	Mitosis and cell differentiation (modulation of microtubule network)
SIRT3	Mitochondria	Deacetylase	Energy metabolism and responses to oxidative stress (ATP level)
SIRT4	Mitochondria	ADP-ribosyltransferase	Energy metabolism and responses to oxidative stress (insulin secretion)
SIRT5	Mitochondria	Deacetylase	Energy metabolism and responses to oxidative stress
SIRT6	Nucleus	ADP-ribosyltransferase, deacetylase	DNA stability and cell proliferation (DNA single-strand break repair)
SIRT7	Nucleus	Deacetylase	DNA stability and cell proliferation

like Sir2, modifies chromatin and silences the transcription of integrated reporter genes via histone deacetylation [15]. In *SIRT1*-deficient embryonic stem cells, oxidative-stress-induced chromosomal fusions, which generally result from aberrantly repaired DNA, are clearly upregulated [4]. On the other hand, SIRT1 overexpression inhibits irradiation-induced cancers, by increasing DNA stability [4]. This result is particularly interesting in view of possible cancer therapies. However, the potential roles of SIRT1 in life span regulation have not yet been documented.

A biological role in aging was reported for SIRT6 [16]. In *SIRT6*-deficient mammalian cells (mouse embryonic fibroblasts and embryonic stem cells), proliferation is reduced, and sensitivity to DNA-damaging agents is increased, as is DNA instability. These events are caused by defective base excision repair, a repair mechanism for DNA single-strand breaks. The *SIRT6*-deficient cells show chromosomal aberrations and genome instability, even in the absence of artificial stimuli. Moreover, *SIRT6*-deficient mice have a reduced life span. This may be due to direct impairment of the base excision repair system; however, these mice also show severely reduced insulin-like growth factor 1 and blood glucose levels, which might also promote DNA instability.

The deacetylase activity of SIRT1 has other substrates besides histones (fig. 1). It also deacetylates p53 (described above), nuclear factor κB (NF-κB) and forkhead transcription factor (FOXO) [6]. Deacetylated NF-κB is easily degraded and has less activity, which inhibits apoptosis. FOXO, a downstream component of insulin signaling, can increase the transcription of both antiapoptotic factors, such as manganese superoxide dismutase (Mn-SOD), and a DNA repair factor, growth-arrest- and DNA-damage-inducible protein 45 (GADD45), and proapoptotic ones, such as B-cell-lymphoma-2-interacting mediator (BIM) and Fas ligand, depending on the context. These different effects can be explained, at least in part, by FOXO regulation by SIRT1. FOXO-induced apoptosis is decreased when SIRT1 is overexpressed in cerebellar neurons [17]. The deacetylation of FOXO by SIRT1 decreases the DNA-binding activity of FOXO and reduces the transcription of apoptotic factors [18]. On the other hand, the association of SIRT1 with FOXO upregulates the expression of antiapoptotic factors. Therefore, SIRT1 uses multiple pathways to modulate cellular resistance to genotoxic stress and apoptosis [13].

SIRT1 protein is mainly localized to the nucleus; however, it can be translocated to the cytoplasm in the presence of oxidative stress, leading to apoptosis [19]. This phenomenon is also observed in *Caenorhabditis elegans* [20]. Sir2.1 translocates from the nucleus to the cytoplasm as an early event of apoptosis, although the causal relationship and the kinetics of this translocation are still obscure.

Therefore, the sirtuins have critical roles in DNA stability and antiapoptotic processes, and they remain key molecules for aging research.

Sirtuins in the Retina

SIRT1 is expressed throughout the retina, including the retinal ganglion cells, inner retinal cells, photoreceptor cells and retinal pigment epithelial cells [21]. *SIRT1*-targeted mice show abnormal retinal development as early as embryonic day 12.5; these abnormalities include persistence of the optic fissure and disorganized retinal morphogenesis, with decreased cellularity in multiple retinal layers [22], although it is not yet known whether these embryonic retinal abnormalities are associated with an increase in p53 expression, as observed in *SIRT1*-targeted mouse embryonic fibroblasts. The deletion of the upstream inducers of SIRT1, E2fs, also cause retinal cell death with the hyperacetylation (i.e. activation) of p53 [23].

SIRT1 activates multiple pathways and has been reported to function in animal models of inflammatory disease. In a multiple sclerosis model of experimental autoimmune encephalomyelitis, the intravitreal injection of SIRT1 activators prevented the death of retinal ganglion cells [24]. This effect was obtained without suppressing the infiltration of inflammatory cells into the optic nerve sheath, suggesting that SIRT1 acted in the retinal ganglion cells themselves.

This successful treatment of ganglion cells is consistent with the result of an experiment using explant neurons of the dorsal root ganglion [25]. Ganglion cell death after axotomy, called wallerian degeneration, is avoided by introduction of nicotinamide mononucleotide adenylyltransferase 1 (Nmnatl), an enzyme in the NAD biosynthesis pathway, which leads to an increase in nuclear NAD. SIRT1 activity induced by a polyphenol compound, resveratrol, has a similar effect. These results indicated that SIRT1, which is NAD dependent, is the effector of the ganglion cell protection conferred by the increased Nmnatl activity and NAD. Moreover, Nmnatl is normally expressed in retinal ganglion cells and their axons [26], which should enable SIRT1 activation in these cells.

A decrease in the deacetylation activity of SIRT1 during retinal inflammation was reported in the endotoxin-induced uveitis model [27]. In this mouse model, 8-oxo-2′-deoxyguanosine (8-OHdG), an oxidized form of deoxyguanosine, a component of DNA, is upregulated, and resveratrol suppresses this upregulation. It would be interesting to examine whether this reduction in DNA oxidation is related to an effect of SIRT1 on DNA and discuss the possible involvement of inflammation in aging.

Role of Sirtuins in the Aging of the Retina

Age-related DNA damage is reported in the rodent retina. An increase in oxidative DNA damage in the 2-year-old retina compared to the 5-month-old retina was shown by 8-OHdG labeling [28]. The authors concluded that this increase in labeling reflected mitochondrial DNA damage resulting from decreased levels of DNA repair enzymes. However, the role of sirtuins in this phenomenon is not addressed.

Abnormal SIRT1 expression is observed in a mutant mouse model of retinal degeneration (*rd* mice) that progresses with age; these *rd* mice have a point mutation in the β-subunit of rod photoreceptor cGMP phosphodiesterase [21]. In the normal mouse retinal ganglion cells, inner nuclear layer cells and a subset of photoreceptors, thought to be cone cells, SIRT1 immunoreactivity appears as granular staining in the nuclei. In the rod photoreceptor cells, it appears as weak peripheral nuclear staining (but is still within the nucleus). However, in the *rd* mice, SIRT1 in the rod photoreceptor cells translocates to the cytoplasm around postnatal day 15, when apoptotic markers (caspase 12 or apoptosis-inducing factor (AIF) as well as transferase-mediated uridine nick end-labeling (TUNEL) staining) become apparent. This finding is consistent with another report that the translocation of SIRT1 protein from the nucleus to the cytoplasm precedes apoptosis in *C. elegans* [20]. The *rd* mutants lose their photoreceptor cells precociously, which is considered an aging phenotype. A similar theory has been proposed to explain brain diseases, such as Parkinson's disease and Alzheimer's disease, in which brain cells degenerate earlier than in the normal life course. Further analyses are required to determine whether the translocation of SIRT1 from the nucleus leads to DNA instability in *rd* mice and in other systems.

In summary, the aging of tissues/organs, including the retina, is caused by accumulated changes that lead to their dysfunction. The fundamental cause is believed to involve DNA instability, which may be induced by extrinsic stimuli, such as light exposure or inflammation, or by intrinsic factors, such as gene abnormalities. The ability of sirtuins to stabilize DNA may, at least in part, determine the progress of aging in the retina.

Acknowledgement

We thank Dr. Susumu Ishida for advice in preparing the manuscript.

References

1 Nakanishi M, Niida H, Murakami H, Shimada M: DNA damage responses in skin biology – implications in tumor prevention and aging acceleration. J Dermatol Sci 2009;56:76–81.

2 Campisi J, Yaswen P: Aging and cancer cell biology, 2009. Aging Cell 2009;8:221–225.

3 Gan L, Mucke L: Paths of convergence: sirtuins in aging and neurodegeneration. Neuron 2008;58:10–14.

4 Oberdoerffer P, Michan S, McVay M, Mostoslavsky R, Vann J, Park SK, Hartlerode A, Stegmuller J, Hafner A, Loerch P, Wright SM, Mills KD, Bonni A, Yankner BA, Scully R, Prolla TA, Alt FW, Sinclair DA: Sirt1 redistribution on chromatin promotes genomic stability but alters gene expression during aging. Cell 2008;135:907–918.

5 Jackson SP: Sensing and repairing DNA double-strand breaks. Carcinogenesis 2002;23:687–696.

6 Niedernhofer LJ, Robbins PD: Signaling mechanisms involved in the response to genotoxic stress and regulating life span. Int J Biochem Cell Biol 2008;40:176–180.

7 Bass TM, Weinkove D, Houthoofd K, Gems D, Partridge L: Effects of resveratrol on lifespan in *Drosophila melanogaster* and *Caenorhabditis elegans*. Mech Ageing Dev 2007;128:546–552.

8 Guarente L, Kenyon C: Genetic pathways that regulate ageing in model organisms. Nature 2000;408:255–262.

9 Finkel T, Deng CX, Mostoslavsky R: Recent progress in the biology and physiology of sirtuins. Nature 2009;460:587–591.

10 Frye RA: Phylogenetic classification of prokaryotic and eukaryotic Sir2-like proteins. Biochem Biophys Res Commun 2000;273:793–798.

11 Haigis MC, Sinclair DA: Mammalian sirtuins: biological insights and disease relevance. Annu Rev Pathol 2010;5:253–295.

12 Haigis MC, Guarente LP: Mammalian sirtuins – emerging roles in physiology, aging, and calorie restriction. Genes Dev 2006;20:2913–2921.

13 Blander G, Guarente L: The Sir2 family of protein deacetylases. Annu Rev Biochem 2004;73:417–435.

14 North BJ, Verdin E: Sirtuins: Sir2-related NAD-dependent protein deacetylases. Genome Biol 2004;5:224.

15 Vaquero A, Scher M, Lee D, Erdjument-Bromage H, Tempst P, Reinberg D: Human SIRT1 interacts with histone H1 and promotes formation of facultative heterochromatin. Mol Cell 2004;16:93–105.

16 Mostoslavsky R, Chua KF, Lombard DB, Pang WW, Fischer MR, Gellon L, Liu P, Mostoslavsky G, Franco S, Murphy MM, Mills KD, Patel P, Hsu JT, Hong AL, Ford E, Cheng HL, Kennedy C, Nunez N, Bronson R, Frendewey D, Auerbach W, Valenzuela D, Karow M, Hottiger MO, Hursting S, Barrett JC, Guarente L, Mulligan R, Demple B, Yancopoulos GD, Alt FW: Genomic instability and aging-like phenotype in the absence of mammalian SIRT6. Cell 2006;124:315–329.

17 Brunet A, Sweeney LB, Sturgill JF, Chua KF, Greer PL, Lin Y, Tran H, Ross SE, Mostoslavsky R, Cohen HY, Hu LS, Cheng HL, Jedrychowski MP, Gygi SP, Sinclair DA, Alt FW, Greenberg ME: Stress-dependent regulation of FOXO transcription factors by the SIRT1 deacetylase. Science 2004;303:2011–2015.

18 Giannakou ME, Partridge L: The interaction between FOXO and SIRT1: tipping the balance towards survival. Trends Cell Biol 2004;14:408–412.

19 Jin Q, Yan T, Ge X, Sun C, Shi X, Zhai Q: Cytoplasm-localized SIRT1 enhances apoptosis. J Cell Physiol 2007;213:88–97.

20 Greiss S, Hall J, Ahmed S, Gartner A: *C. elegans* SIR-2.1 translocation is linked to a proapoptotic pathway parallel to cep-1/p53 during DNA damage-induced apoptosis. Genes Dev 2008;22:2831–2842.

21 Jaliffa C, Ameqrane I, Dansault A, Leemput J, Vieira V, Lacassagne E, Provost A, Bigot K, Masson C, Menasche M, Abitbol M: Sirt1 involvement in rd10 mouse retinal degeneration. Invest Ophthalmol Vis Sci 2009;50:3562–3572.

22 Cheng HL, Mostoslavsky R, Saito S, Manis JP, Gu Y, Patel P, Bronson R, Appella E, Alt FW, Chua KF: Developmental defects and p53 hyperacetylation in Sir2 homolog (SIRT1)-deficient mice. Proc Natl Acad Sci USA 2003;100:10794–10799.

23 Chen D, Pacal M, Wenzel P, Knoepfler PS, Leone G, Bremner R: Division and apoptosis of E2f-deficient retinal progenitors. Nature 2009;462:925–929.

24 Shindler KS, Ventura E, Rex TS, Elliott P, Rostami A: SIRT1 activation confers neuroprotection in experimental optic neuritis. Invest Ophthalmol Vis Sci 2007;48:3602–3609.

25 Araki T, Sasaki Y, Milbrandt J: Increased nuclear NAD biosynthesis and SIRT1 activation prevent axonal degeneration. Science 2004;305:1010–1013.

26 Kitaoka Y, Hayashi Y, Kumai T, Takeda H, Munemasa Y, Fujino H, Kitaoka Y, Ueno S, Sadun AA, Lam TT: Axonal and cell body protection by nicotinamide adenine dinucleotide in tumor necrosis factor-induced optic neuropathy. J Neuropathol Exp Neurol 2009;68:915–927.

27 Kubota S, Kurihara T, Mochimaru H, Satofuka S, Noda K, Ozawa Y, Oike Y, Ishida S, Tsubota K: Prevention of ocular inflammation in endotoxin-induced uveitis with resveratrol by inhibiting oxidative damage and nuclear factor-kappaB activation. Invest Ophthalmol Vis Sci 2009;50:3512–3519.

28 Wang AL, Lukas TJ, Yuan M, Neufeld AH: Age-related increase in mitochondrial DNA damage and loss of DNA repair capacity in the neural retina. Neurobiol Aging, E-pub ahead of print.

Ophthalmic Research

Author Index Vol. 44, No. 3, 2010

Subject Index Vol. 44, No. 3, 2010

KARGER
Fax +41 61 306 12 34
E-Mail karger@karger.ch
www.karger.com

Accessible online at:
www.karger.com/ore